A Pocket Guide
to Respiratory Disease

A Pocket Guide to Respiratory Disease

Robert L. Wilkins, PhD, RRT, FAARC
Professor and Chair
Department of Cardiopulmonary Sciences
School of Allied Health Professions
Loma Linda University
Loma Linda, California

Thomas J. Butler, MS, RRT, RPFT
Associate Professor
Allied Health
SUNY Rockland Community College
Suffern, New York
and
Respiratory Care Manager
Kessler Institute for Rehabilitation
West Orange, New Jersey

James R. Dexter, MD
Associate Clinical Professor
School of Medicine
Loma Linda University
Loma Linda, California
and
Medical Director
Department of Respiratory Care
Redlands Community Hospital
Redlands, California

 F. A. DAVIS COMPANY • Philadelphia

F. A. Davis Company
1915 Arch Street
Philadelphia, PA 19103
www.fadavis.com

Copyright © 2001 by F.A. Davis Company

Printed in Canada

Last digit indicates print number: 10 9 8 7 6 5 4 3

Acquisitions Editor: Lynn Borders Caldwell
Developmental Editor: Margaret Biblis
Production Editor: Jessica Howie Martin
Cover Designer: Louis J. Forgione

As new scientific information becomes available through basic and clinical research, recommended treatments and drug therapies undergo changes. The authors and publisher have done everything possible to make this book accurate, up to date, and in accord with accepted standards at the time of publication. The authors, editors, and publisher are not responsible for errors or omissions or for consequences from application of the book, and make no warranty, expressed or implied, in regard to the contents of the book. Any practice described in this book should be applied by the reader in accordance with professional standards of care used in regard to the unique circumstances that may apply in each situation. The reader is advised always to check product information (package inserts) for changes and new information regarding dose and contraindications before administering any drug. Caution is especially urged when using new or infrequently ordered drugs.

Library of Congress Cataloging-in-Publication Data

Wilkins, Robert L.
A pocket guide to respiratory disease / Robert L. Wilkins, Thomas J. Butler, James R. Dexter.
p. cm.
Includes bibliographical references.
ISBN 0-8036-0566-8 (pbk.)
1. Respiratory organs—Diseases—Handbooks, manuals, etc. I. Butler, Thomas J. II. Dexter, James R., 1948– III. Title.
RC732.W55 2001
616.2—dc21   2001017288

DEDICATION

We would like to dedicate this book to all the graduates of the SUNY Rockland Community College and the Loma Linda University Respiratory Care programs. Over the years, their enthusiasm and hard work challenged us to provide the best possible learning experience. We can only hope that we inspired them as much!

HOW TO USE THIS BOOK

 This pocket guide, which is based on the student textbook, *Respiratory Disease: A Case Study Approach to Patient Care, 2nd edition*, provides the bedside clinician and student with a concise, accurate, and current overview of key Information related to the assessment and treatment of patients with cardiopulmonary disease. Respiratory therapists are often called on to assess a patient at the bedside and suggest appropriate treatment. This book will help the respiratory therapist provide accurate patient assessments and rapid and accurate treatment.

The diseases are listed alphabetically, and each chapter follows the same format. Key terms; epidemiology and etiology; clinical features including history, physical examination and laboratory data; and treatment are included for each disease. This provides the clinician with a brief trend or pattern of the disease to help differentiate one disease from another and formulate the best treatment plan. If more in-depth information is needed, readers should consult the complete textbook on which this pocket guide is based or one of the many comprehensive textbooks available.

We have included a list of Questions Frequently Asked by Patient or Caregiver in each chapter, along with possible responses to these questions. We believe that our suggested responses will help educate patients about their diseases and treatment options. Questions that require a definitive answer about treatment, test results, and prognosis should be considered carefully and referred to the attending physician when appropriate.

Robert L. Wilkins
Thomas J. Butler
James R. Dexter

ACKNOWLEDGMENTS

We would especially like to thank Dr. Lennard Specht for his assistance in providing information to strengthen selected chapters. His input proved to be most valuable.

We also thank Larry Totaro, RRT; Anna Cameron, RRT; Kelly Matzen, RRT; and Edward Rajah, RRT for contributing some of the Questions Frequently Asked by Patient or Caregiver and the following people for reviewing the manuscript and providing valuable feedback:

Charles S. Cornfield, MS, RRT
Program Director
Department of Respiratory Care
Gannon University
Erie, Pennsylvania

William F. Galvin, MSEd, RRT, CPFT
Assistant Professor
School of Allied Health Professions
Program Director
Respiratory Care Program
Gwynedd Mercy College
Gwynedd Valley, Pennsylvania

Brian Kellar MS, RRT, RPFT
Clinical Educator
Respiratory Care Services
Jefferson Health System—Main Line
Bryn Mawr, Pennsylvania

Sam Gregory Marshall, PhD, RRT, RCP
Associate Professor
Department of Respiratory Therapy
Southwest Texas State University
San Marcos, Texas

Robert G. McGee, MSEd, RRT
Associate Professor
Department of Respiratory Therapy
Walters State Community College
Greenville, Tennessee

Marta Lee Tingdale, RRT, RN
Manager
Department of Pulmonary Services
Baylor University Medical Center
Dallas, Texas

CONTENTS

ABBREVIATIONS USED IN THIS BOOK

ABG	arterial blood gas
AIDS	acquired immunodeficiency syndrome
ALS	amyotrophic lateral sclerosis
A-P	anteroposterior
ARDS	acute respiratory distress syndrome
BCG	bacillus Calmette-Guerin
BP	blood pressure
BPD	bronchopulmonary dysplasia
CAD	coronary artery disease
C&S	culture and sensitivity
CBC	complete blood count
CF	cystic fibrosis
CHF	congestive heart failure
CMV	cytomegalovirus
CNS	central nervous system
CO	carbon monoxide
COPD	chronic obstructive pulmonary disease
CPAP	continuous positive airway pressure
CPR	cardiopulmonary resuscitation
CT	computed tomography
DLCO	carbon monoxide diffusing capacity
ECG	electrocardiogram
ECMO	extracorporeal membrane oxygenation
EMS	emergency medical service
ER	emergency room
FEV_1	forced expiratory volume in one second
FIO_2	fraction of inspired gas made up of oxygen
FVC	forced vital capacity

ABBREVIATIONS USED IN THIS BOOK

HEENT	head, eyes, ears, nose, throat
HF	heart failure
HIV	human immunodeficiency virus
HR	heart rate
IBW	ideal body weight
ICU	intensive care unit
IM	intramuscular
INH	isoniazid
IPPB	intermittent positive pressure breathing
IV	intravenous
IVH	intravascular hemorrhage
JVD	jugular venous distention
LMWH	low molecular weight heparin
MD	muscular dystrophy
MDI	metered-dose inhaler
MRI	magnetic resonance imaging
MS	multiple sclerosis
MSLT	multiple sleep latency test
NICU	neonatal intensive care unit
NREM	non–rapid eye movement
OSA	obstructive sleep apnea
PCWP	pulmonary capillary wedge pressure
PDA	patent ductus arteriosus
PEEP	positive end-expiratory pressure
PFC	persistent fetal circulation
PFT	pulmonary function test
PIP	peak inspiratory pressure
PMI	point of maximal impulse

ABBREVIATIONS USED IN THIS BOOK

PPD	purified protein derivative
PPHN	persistent pulmonary hypertension of the newborn
PPV	positive-pressure ventilation
RBC	red blood cell
RDS	respiratory distress syndrome
REM	rapid eye movement
RSV	respiratory syncytial virus
SK	streptokinase
SIDS	sudden infant death syndrome
SOB	shortness of breath
SPAG	small particle aerosol generator
SVN	small-volume nebulizer
SVR	systemic vascular resistance
TB	tuberculosis
TLC	total lung capacity
TTN	transient tachypnea of the newborn
UPPP	uvulopalatopharyngoplasty
VAP	ventilator-associated pneumonia
VC	ventilatory capacity
V/P	ventilation/perfusion
WBC	white blood cell count

Chapter 1

Bedside Patient Assessment

The purpose of this chapter is to provide you with reminders of how to assess a patient with cardiopulmonary disease at the bedside. Techniques of interviewing, physical examination, and interpretation of common laboratory tests are reviewed. The final section of this chapter includes frequently asked questions (FAQs) from patients to the examiner during the assessment process.

KEY TERMS

abdominal paradox–abnormal inward movement of the abdomen with each inspiratory effort

adventitious lung sounds–abnormal lung sound superimposed on the breath sounds (e.g., crackles or wheezes)

anemia–abnormal decrease in RBC count

barrel chest–abnormal increase in the AP diameter of the chest

bradycardia–abnormally low heart rate

breath sounds–the normal sounds of breathing

bronchial breath sounds–abnormal tubular type of breath sounds heard over the peripheral chest

cyanosis–abnormal bluish discoloration of the skin or mucous membranes caused by hypoxemia

digital clubbing–abnormal enlargement of the distal portion of the fingers

dyspnea–labored or difficult breathing

fever–elevated body temperature caused by disease

heave–abnormal pulsation felt over the precordium

hemoptysis–coughing up bloody sputum

hypotension–abnormally low blood pressure

hypoxemia–PaO_2 below the expected normal range

kyphoscoliosis–abnormal lateral and AP curvature of the spine

kyphosis–abnormal AP curvature of the spine

leukocytosis–abnormal elevation of the WBC count

monophonic wheeze–single-note wheeze

mucoid sputum–thick but clear sputum

orthopnea–improved breathing in the upright position

pectus carinatum–abnormal and permanent protrusion of the sternum

pectus excavatum–abnormal and permanent depression of the sternum

platypnea–shortness of breath in the upright position

polycythemia–abnormally high RBC count

polyphonic wheezing–wheezing with multiple musical-type notes beginning and ending at the same time

purulent sputum–sputum containing pus

retractions–abnormal breathing pattern in which the skin around the ribs sinks inward with each inspiratory effort

rhonchi–low-pitched continuous adventitious lung sound

scoliosis–abnormal lateral curvature of the spine

sensorium–orientation to time, place, and person

stridor–abnormal monophonic wheeze emanating from the upper airway

tachycardia–abnormally elevated heart rate

tachypnea–elevated breathing rate

tactile fremitus–vibrations felt over the chest wall as the patient repeats a phrase such as "99" (increased tactile fremitus is associated with lung consolidation)

wheeze–continuous type of adventitious lung sound with a musical quality

INTERVIEWING AND THE MEDICAL HISTORY

Ask questions to clarify the following about each new symptom:

- What seemed to provoke it?
- When did it start?
- How severe is it?
- Have you had this before? If so, how does this episode compare with others?
- Where exactly is the pain?
- Does anything seem to make the symptoms worse or better?
- Are you taking any medications for the problem?

COMMON SYMPTOMS IN PATIENTS WITH CARDIOPULMONARY DISEASE

- Shortness of breath (intensity, duration, quality)
- Cough (frequency, productivity, strength, associated pain)
- Sputum production (quantity, color, viscosity)
- Chest pain (intensity, location, quality)
- Wheezing
- Fever (time of day, measured versus subjective sensation, intensity)
- Night sweats (intensity, time of day)

COMMON FORMAT FOR REPORTING THE MEDICAL HISTORY

- Patient identification
- History of present illness
- Review of systems

- Past medical history
- Past surgical history
- Current medications
- Allergies
- Social history
- Family history

PHYSICAL EXAMINATION

Vital Signs

Table 1–1 lists the normal range for vital signs and causes of deviation from normal.

Inspection

Breathing Pattern

- Note any use of accessory muscles to breathe.
- Prolonged expiratory time suggests intrathoracic airway obstruction (e.g., asthma).
- Prolonged inspiratory time suggests extrathoracic airway obstruction (e.g., croup).
- Abdominal paradox suggests diaphragm fatigue.
- Note any pursed-lipped breathing.
- Note digital clubbing.
- Note any evidence of previous chest surgery.

Color of Mucous Membranes

- Cyanosis of the oral mucosa suggests central cyanosis and respiratory failure.

Chest Configuration

- Large AP diameter is consistent with a barrel chest and emphysema.
- Lateral curvature of the spine is scoliosis.
- AP curvature of the spine is kyphosis.

Palpation

Tactile Fremitus

- Increased with lung consolidation
- Decreased with pneumothorax and lung hyperinflation

Table 1–1 *Vital Signs*

Parameter	Normal Range	Causes of Deviation from Normal
Respiratory rate	12–18/min	Increased with atelectasis, fever, anxiety, and as a side effect of certain medications; decreased with hypothermia and brain injury
Heart rate	60–100/min	Increased with hypoxemia, anxiety, pain, fever; decreased with hypothermia, heart disease
Body temperature	36.5–37.5°C (98–99.5°F)	Increased with infection such as pneumonia; decreased with hypothermia and certain brain injuries
Blood pressure	90–140/ 60–90 mm Hg	Increased with stress, vasoconstriction; decreased with shock, heart disease, hypovolemia
Sensorium	Oriented × 3	Normal when the patient is oriented to time, place, and person; becomes abnormal when the brain is not well oxygenated

Skin Temperature

- Cool extremities suggest poor circulation.
- Capillary refill (normal <3 sec; >3 sec suggests poor circulation).

Percussion

Lung Resonance

- Increased with pneumothorax and lung hyperinflation
- Decreased with lung consolidation and pleural effusion

Position of Diaphragm

- Elevated with severe atelectasis
- Low and flat with severe emphysema

Auscultation

Breath Sounds

- Diminished with lung hyperinflation, mucus plugging, and shallow breathing
- Increased with lung consolidation and atelectasis

Adventitious Lung Sounds

- Fine, late-inspiratory crackles suggest restrictive lung disease (e.g., atelectasis or pulmonary fibrosis).
- Early inspiratory crackles are consistent with COPD.
- Polyphonic expiratory wheezing is consistent with bronchitis or asthma.
- Monophonic wheezing indicates narrowing of a single airway.

LABORATORY DATA

Complete Blood Count

- Normal WBC count is about 4500 to 9500 cells/mm^3.
- Elevated WBC count (leukocytosis) is consistent with infection, stress, other diseases.
- Decreased WBC count (leukopenia) is consistent with overwhelming infection or bone marrow disease.
- Elevated neutrophil count on the differential is consistent with bacterial infection.
- Elevated eosinophil count on the differential is consistent with an allergic reaction.
- Elevated lymphocyte count on the differential is consistent with a viral infection.

- Normal RBC count is about 3 to 5 million cells/mm^3; normal hemoglobin is about 12 to 15 g/mL.
- Elevated RBC count (polycythemia) is often caused by chronic hypoxemia.
- Decreased RBC count (anemia) is consistent with blood loss or bone marrow disease.

Sputum Gram Stain

- Legitimate sputum sample has few epithelial cells and numerous pus cells.
- Presence of many pus cells is consistent with an infection in the lung or airways.

Sputum culture identifies the specific organism responsible for the infection.

ABG

Steps to Interpretation of an ABG

- Look at the PaO$_2$ (<40 mm Hg=severe hypoxemia; 41 to 59 mm Hg=moderate hypoxemia; 59 to 79 mm Hg=mild hypoxemia).
- Assess acid-base status; pH <7.35=acidosis, pH >7.45=alkalosis.
- Elevated PCO$_2$ is consistent with respiratory acidosis.
- HCO$_3$ <22 mEq/L is consistent with metabolic acidosis.
- PCO$_2$ below the predicted level=respiratory alkalosis.
- HCO$_3$ above the predicted level=metabolic alkalosis.

Pulmonary Function Data

- Obstructive pattern seen as reduced expiratory flow rates (peak flow <300 to 400 L/min, FEV$_1$/FVC below 75%); evidence of air trapping also common (increase residual volume)
- Restrictive pattern seen as reduced lung volumes; VC <80% of predicted; TLC <80% of predicted; FEV$_1$/FVC normal with pure restrictive defect

ECG

Steps to Review of the ECG Tracing

- Determine the atrial and ventricular rates.

- Measure the P-R interval (should be <0.20 sec).
- Measure the QRS interval (<0.12 sec).
- Inspect the S-T segment for elevation or depression (elevated S-T segment is consistent with myocardial ischemia).
- Examine the T wave for contour (inverted T waves=ischemia).
- Look for evidence of right-axis deviation (negative QRS in lead I).

Chest Radiograph

Steps to Interpretation of the Chest Radiograph

- Examine the heart size and location (heart shadow should not be more than one half the width of the chest).
- Examine the tracheal air shadow for position (should overlap the spinous processes of the vertebral column).
- Examine the hilum for location.
- Inspect the lung fields for areas of consolidation or hyperinflation.
- Examine the bony structures for evidence of fracture.
- Inspect the soft tissues around the chest for evidence of trauma.
- Inspect the costophrenic angles for sharpness; blunted angles suggest pleural effusion.
- Evaluate the position of the diaphragm (the 8 to 10 posterior ribs are normally visible above the diaphragm at full inspiration).

QUESTIONS FREQUENTLY ASKED BY PATIENT OR CAREGIVER

1. Why do the nurses and doctors often ask if I know my name, where I am, and the date?

Many illnesses can make the blood levels of oxygen in the brain drop too low. This may cause you to temporarily lose track of time, place, and who you are. Periodic checks of this information helps us determine whether you are getting better or having any side effects. Other problems in addition to low oxygen levels in the blood also cause change in orientation, so finding trends in this information is important in many circumstances.

2. Can having several chest x-rays be harmful and increase my risk of lung cancer?

It would be very unusual for chest x-rays to cause a problem because there is so little radiation emitted from the x-ray machine (about the same as a day at the beach). However, if you could be pregnant, be sure to tell your doctor and have the radiation technician place a lead shield over your abdomen.

3. Why does everyone listen to my chest when they evaluate me?

Air moving in and out of your chest makes noise. By listening carefully to each lobe of the lung, we can determine how much each portion of your lung is participating in gas exchange. We are also listening for abnormal sounds, such as wheezes or crackles, that occur when certain illnesses are present.

4. Why did the doctor ask about my smoking history when I am here to have abdominal surgery?

Abdominal surgery is done near the diaphragm and reduces lung function for several weeks after the surgery. Smokers are at higher risk for postoperative pulmonary complications, especially if they are not treated with bronchial hygiene and have stopped smoking at least 5 days before the surgery.

5. Why did the doctor want to know about my recent traveling outside the United States and to certain regions around this country?

Some illnesses are common only in specific parts of the world. For example, coccidioidomycosis is seen primarily in southern California and Arizona; histoplasmosis is seen in the Ohio River Valley; and *Pseudomonas pseudomallei* infection is found in Southeast Asia.

6. Why did the doctor want to know about the color of my sputum and whether there was any blood in it?

The color of your sputum may provide clues about what is going on in your lungs and airways. For example, clear sputum is often associated with allergies. Green or yellow sputum can also occur with allergies but may be a sign of infection. Blood in your sputum is not usually serious, but your doctor wants to know whether other tests may be needed and the presence of blood may help the doctor narrow down the list of possible illnesses causing your illness.

7. Why did the doctor ask whether I could walk up a flight of stairs without stopping to catch my breath?

An easy screening for lung disease is exercise tolerance. If you can walk up a flight of stairs without shortness of breath, severe lung disease is not likely.

8. Why did my doctor ask about night sweats?

Some patients have mild to moderate fever but are not aware of it. When such a fever "breaks" in the middle of the night, the patient often has night sweats as his or her body adjusts to a lower temperature. The complaint of night sweats tells your doctor that you may be experiencing fevers.

9. Why is my pulse rate so fast?

Many types of illnesses and stresses can increase your heart rate. It is more important to know how fast your heart is beating, for how long, and whether it is regular. Don't worry about it because in most cases the heart rate comes down to normal range when the underlying illness or disease is treated.

10. Why are my fingers blue at times?

Low oxygen levels in the blood cause blood to turn dark blue. Cold can also make your fingers appear a little blue.

11. Does having chest pain mean that I am having a heart attack?

Not necessarily. Some chest pain is related to inflammation of the lung or other organs in the chest. However, if the chest pain is centrally located and radiates to your arm or back, you should seek medical attention immediately because these are signs of heart attack.

Reference

Wilkins, RL, and Dexter, JR: Respiratory Disease: A Case Study Approach to Patient Care, second edition. FA Davis, Philadelphia, 1998.

Chapter 2

Adult Respiratory Distress Syndrome

ARDS is hypoxemic respiratory failure caused by damage to the alveolar capillary membrane that leads to diffuse pulmonary edema. The lungs become difficult to expand, and poor oxygenation is a serious threat to life. ARDS is often accompanied by failure of other organ systems.

KEY TERMS

optimal PEEP–the level of PEEP that results in the best PaO_2 without decreasing cardiac output

permissive hypercapnia–the use of tidal volumes below normal during mechanical ventilation, which allows the $PaCO_2$ to rise above normal, decreasing mean airway pressure to minimize the risk of pulmonary barotrauma

protective lung ventilation–strategies used during mechanical ventilation to reduce the risk of barotrauma; these include pressure control ventilation and ventilating in the prone position

refractory hypoxemia–persistent low levels of PaO_2 despite significant increases in FIO_2

right-to-left shunt–blood passing through the lung without exposure to oxygenated alveoli

shock lung–another term used to describe ARDS

static compliance–volume change per unit of applied pressure under conditions of no flow

EPIDEMIOLOGY

Approximately 150,000 cases occur each year in the United States.

ETIOLOGY

Frequent causes include:

- Shock with persistent low blood pressure
- Chest trauma
- Systemic infection (sepsis)
- Aspiration
- Inhalation injury
- Postoperative for major surgery

CLINICAL FEATURES

Medical History

Chief Complaints

Sudden onset of dyspnea with labored breathing. Patient usually denies cough or sputum production.

History of Present Illness

The patient has a recent history of trauma or some catastrophic event within the past 48 hours or has been diagnosed with sepsis. The patient has a rapid onset of labored and rapid breathing despite an increase in FIO_2 (refractory hypoxemia).

Past Medical History

Noncontributory to the diagnosis but may influence the patient's ability to tolerate the respiratory failure.

Family History

Noncontributory.

Allergies

None.

Physical Examination

- Diminished orientation to time, place, and person. Tachypnea and tachycardia are present. Blood pressure is often normal or low. Body temperature is usually normal unless an infection is present.
- **HEENT:** Cyanosis of the oral mucosa may be present.
- **Neck:** Use of accessory muscles.

- **Chest:** Fine inspiratory crackles in both lungs; retractions with rapid and shallow breathing are common before intubation and mechanical ventilation.
- **Abdomen:** Noncontributory.
- **Extremities:** Noncontributory, although cyanosis may be present.

Laboratory Data

- **ABG:** Demonstrates persistent hypoxemia despite elevation of the FIO_2. Hypercapnia is not common, at least in the early stages of the syndrome.
- **CBC:** Often normal unless an infection is present.
- **Chest radiography:** Diffuse fluffy infiltrates with normal heart size.
- **PCWP:** Usually normal or low (<16 mm Hg).
- **PaO_2/FIO_2 ratio:** <200.

TREATMENT

Treatment is supportive until the precipitating factor is treated and the patient has time to recover.

- Mechanical ventilation with PEEP and an FIO_2 to keep the PaO_2 60 to 80 mm Hg. Permissive hypercapnia may be used to avoid barotrauma. Mechanical tidal volumes in the range of 5 to 7 mL/kg are often used.
- Antibiotics may be needed if infection is present.
- Vasopressors may be needed if blood pressure is persistently low.

Figure 2–1 outlines the assessment and treatment of pulmonary edema, the major manifestation of ARDS.

QUESTIONS FREQUENTLY ASKED BY PATIENT OR CAREGIVER

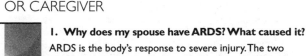

1. Why does my spouse have ARDS? What caused it?

ARDS is the body's response to severe injury. The two most common types of injury that result in ARDS are severe trauma such as an automobile accident with blood loss and low blood pressure and infection severe enough to cause shock with low blood pressure.

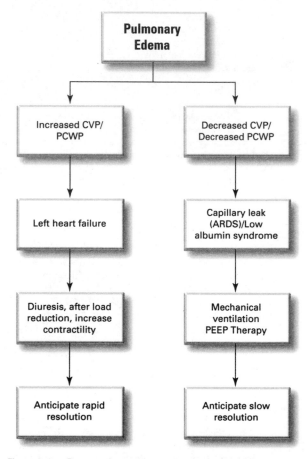

Figure 2–1. *Presentation and treatment of pulmonary edema.*

2. How does the doctor know that my spouse has ARDS?

Extra fluid in the lungs makes them stiff and difficult to expand. This fluid also impairs oxygenation of the blood by the lungs. Stiff lungs are difficult to inflate, so your spouse will have rapid and shallow breathing and poor oxygenation during the early stages. The fluid shows up on the chest radiograph as white shadows. The combination of white shadows on the chest radiograph, poor oxygenation of the blood, and rapid and shallow breathing in a patient with a recent history of trauma points toward the diagnosis of ARDS.

3. What does ARDS do to the lungs?

Severe injury with hypotension triggers a series of events that causes the blood vessels in the lungs to leak fluid into the alveoli and other tissues of the lungs that normally do not have fluid in them. This causes severe respiratory failure that is difficult to treat.

4. How long does the disease last?

The acute phase of the disease usually requires mechanical ventilation for 1 to 3 weeks. The process then slowly improves over the next several weeks.

5. Will my spouse have to carry an oxygen tank around for the rest of his or her life?

Probably not. A total of 50% to 70% of patients with ARDS survive, and those that do survive usually return to near-normal lung function within 6 months of recovery.

6. Why can't my spouse move or respond to me?

A patient's breathing must be carefully controlled during the acute phase of the respiratory failure. Most patients do better if they are given a medication that causes temporary paralysis of the body and allows complete control of their ventilation during the acute phase of the problem. This medication that causes temporary paralysis will be discontinued in a few days when the patient's lungs have improved.

7. Does my spouse know what is happening, or is he or she having pain?

The paralyzing agent is accompanied with pain medication and sedatives, so your spouse should be very relaxed and not feel any pain. It is good for you to talk to your spouse and encourage him or her because he or she may be able to fully understand what you are saying.

8. Will my spouse remember all that happened to him or her here in the ICU?

Our experience is that most patients who are sick enough to be mechanically ventilated for days and then recover have a blank spot in their memory for most of the hospitalization. The blank period usually diminishes with time, but the memory is rarely recovered. There may be one or two vivid memories from the ICU experience, but even that is unusual.

9. How can you tell if my spouse's lungs are getting worse or better?

The easiest way is for us to look at how much oxygen is needed to maintain adequate levels in the body. The trends in ventilatory and oxygen requirements are most useful.

10. What treatments are available for ARDS?

No specific treatment is available. The key to survival is meticulous attention to detail with ventilatory support, nutrition, fluid and electrolyte balance, appropriate antibiotic therapy, and so on. Such support is needed until the lungs have time to heal on their own.

Reference

Wilkins, RL, and Dexter, JR: Respiratory Disease: A Case Study Approach to Patient Care, second edition. FA Davis, Philadelphia, 1998.

Chapter 3

Asthma

Asthma is a type of COPD characterized by diffuse airway inflammation and bronchospasm that, in many cases, occurs in response to various stimuli. A key feature of asthma is reversible airway obstruction. Some common terms associated with asthma are listed below.

KEY TERMS

exercise-induced asthma–condition characterized by a history of asthma with increased symptoms in response to exercise

extrinsic asthma–asthma caused by allergic reactions

intrinsic asthma–asthma in a patient with no evidence of an allergic component

nocturnal asthma–asthma with increased symptoms during sleep

occupational asthma–asthma attacks that occur only when the patient is exposed to specific stimuli in the workplace

pulsus paradoxus–a significant decrease in the pulse pressure with each inspiratory effort

rescue medications–medications designed to provide rapid relief from dyspnea in asthmatic patients during acute asthma attacks

status asthmaticus–a severe asthma attack unresponsive to conventional treatment

stable asthma–type of asthma in a patient with a history of asthma who has not had an increase in symptoms over the past 4 weeks

unstable asthma–type of asthma in a patient with a history of asthma who has had an increase in symptoms or an increased need for medication during the past 4 weeks

EPIDEMIOLOGY

- Approximately 10 million Americans have asthma.
- About two thirds of those with asthma are children under the age of 18 years.
- Approximately 4.1 people per 100 in the U.S. have asthma.
- The rate for children increases to about 5.7 per 100.

ETIOLOGY

Possible triggers of an asthma attack include:

- Respiratory infection
- Dusts
- Pollens
- Animal dander
- Strong fumes or odors
- Occupationally related fumes, vapors, gases, or aerosols
- Medications such as aspirin or beta-blockers
- Exercise
- Cigarette smoke
- Food additives
- Emotional stress
- Changes in weather

CLINICAL FEATURES

Medical History

Chief Complaints

Episodic dyspnea and cough

History of Present Illness

Patient often presents with a recent history of upper respiratory tract infection. Sudden onset of dyspnea, wheezing, and cough may occur.

Past Medical History

The patient often has allergic disorders such as eczema.

Family History

Family members often have asthma or allergic disorders.

Physical Examination

- Rapid pulse and respiratory rate; sensorium normal initially but deteriorates with hypoxia; paradoxical pulse common with more severe cases.
- Prolonged expiratory phase and polyphonic expiratory wheezing.
- Heavy use of accessory muscles common.
- Retractions may be seen with more severe cases.
- Cyanosis may be present.

Laboratory Data

ABG: Moderate to severe hypoxemia; respiratory alkalosis initially; may progress to respiratory acidosis.

CBC: Elevated eosinophil count common; WBC count elevated with infection.

PFT: Reduced FEV_1, peak flow, and vital capacity; increased TLC and RV.

Chest radiograph: Normal with mild to moderate exacerbations; hyperinflation noted with more severe cases; evidence of pneumonia or pneumothorax should be noted.

TREATMENT

Two goals should be kept in mind during treatment of a patient who is experiencing an acute asthma attack:

1. Correction of hypoxemia with oxygen therapy
2. Reduction of airway inflammation and bronchospasm
   - Give oxygen in sufficient amounts to increase the PaO_2 in the 80 to 100 mm Hg range. This can be accomplished with a simple mask or nasal cannula in most cases. In more severe cases, a non-rebreathing mask may be needed.

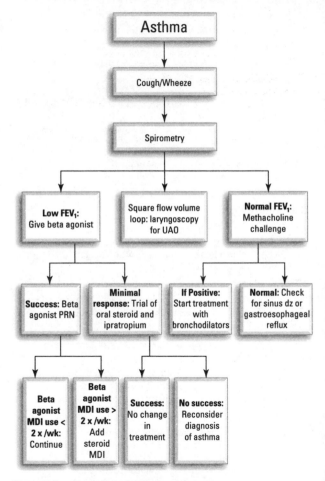

Figure 3–1. *Treatment of asthma.*

- Airway obstruction is reduced by the application of pharmacologic agents. The first line of treatment is the use of beta-adrenergic bronchodilators such as albuterol. These medications can be given by an MDI or by use of small volume nebulizer. MDI is less labor intensive, but the small-volume nebulizer offers humidity therapy.
- The second line of pharmacologic agents useful in the treatment of acute asthma are corticosteroids such as methylprednisolone or hydrocortisone.
- An anticholinergic can be added if the beta-adrenergic bronchodilator and corticosteroids are not effective enough to significantly reduce symptoms. The most common anticholinergic agent applied in this setting is ipratropium bromide.
- Hydration of the patient is often needed and is an important part of treatment in any severe case of asthma. Antibiotics may be needed if bacterial infection is present. Intubation and mechanical ventilation are needed when evidence of respiratory failure is present (e.g., increasing $PaCO_2$ or severe hypoxemia despite an $FIO_2 > 0.60$). If the PCO_2 increases to the point that it crosses over the PO_2 and becomes higher than the PO_2, the patient probably needs intubation and mechanical ventilation.
- Evidence that the asthma patient may need intubation and mechanical ventilation includes:
  - Abnormal sensorium
  - Increasing $PaCO_2$
  - Abdominal paradox present
  - Poor response to maximum therapy
  - Metabolic acidosis seen on ABG even after therapy given
- After the patient is stable, efforts should be made to identify triggers and prevent future attacks or at least minimize their severity.

Figure 3–1 outlines the treatment of asthma.

QUESTIONS FREQUENTLY ASKED BY PATIENT OR CAREGIVER

1. At what peak flow level should I call my doctor?

A good rule of thumb is to call your doctor if your peak flow reduces to less than 50% of your personal best.

2. How can I tell how much medication is left in the MDI canister?

Float it in water. If it floats lying flat on the water, it is empty. If it floats vertically in the water, it is full.

3. Why is my breathing so noisy?

Your airways are narrowed and congested with mucus. Moving air with breathing through these airways causes turbulent airflow and added sounds.

4. Will this medication cause any long-term side effects?

Oral steroids are associated with weight gain, diabetes, cataracts, thin skin, and bruising. All other medications are safe, even in pregnancy. You should consult your physician to clarify the details.

5. Is there a cure for my asthma?

There is no cure, but treatment is usually very effective.

6. Will my asthma get better when I get through puberty?

Often childhood asthma does improve during puberty. However, some asthma patients may experience a return of symptoms later during adulthood.

7. Which is better, the MDI treatment or the small-volume nebulizer treatment?

MDI is easier to use; SVN is better only if the patient is unable to coordinate squeezing the MDI and breathing. MDI is much more portable.

8. If I have children, will they also have asthma?

There is no direct genetic link. Children of asthmatic patients are slightly more likely than normal to have asthma, but no one can predict the odds of your children also having asthma.

9. Should I wear a bracelet that tells others I have asthma?

Most patients with asthma have mild disease and do not need such a bracelet unless they are highly allergic to certain medications or foods. Only those with more severe disease who are prone to acute respiratory failure need to wear such a bracelet.

10. Why do I cough so much?

Asthma causes airway inflammation and mucus production. These two elements combine to trigger cough mechanisms in the airways.

11. Will I need an oxygen bottle when I get older?

No, not unless another lung problem develops in addition to your asthma.

12. Why do I need two MDIs?

One is used as a rescue medication to help with acute episodes of shortness of breath. The other is useful to reduce inflammation in the airways on a long-term basis.

13. Should I continue to take my medication even when I feel well?

Yes, but you can reduce or stop taking certain ones, such as those designated as "rescue meds." Ask your doctor for specific details.

Reference

Wilkins, RL, and Dexter, JR: Respiratory Disease: A Case Study Approach to Patient Care, second edition. FA Davis, Philadelphia, 1998.

Chapter 4

Atelectasis

Atelectasis is a collapsed or airless condition of the lung. It can be caused by a variety of conditions. The amount of lung involved determines the degree of impairment in gas exchange.

KEY TERMS

air bronchogram–an abnormal finding on the chest radiograph seen as dark streaks of air caused by air filled airways surrounded by consolidated lung tissue; often seen in patients with atelectasis

bronchial hygiene therapy–a combination of humidity and aerosol therapy with clapping and postural drainage for the purpose of removing excessive lung secretions

incentive spirometry–a lung expansion technique that encourages the patient prone to atelectasis (through visual cues) to periodically breathe deeply

lobar atelectasis–collapse of a specific lobe of the lung

microatelectasis–a diffuse pattern of atelectasis

passive atelectasis–atelectasis caused by persistent breathing with small tidal volumes

reabsorption atelectasis–atelectasis caused by mucus blockage of a distal airway; gas distal to the blockage is absorbed into the blood, resulting in atelectasis

surfactant–a substance produced by the lung to lower surface tension; pulmonary surfactant is a phospholipid substance that helps prevent alveolar collapse

ETIOLOGY

Factors associated with an increased risk for atelectasis include:

- General anesthesia
- Obesity
- Prolonged bedrest
- Abdominal or thoracic surgery
- Neuromuscular disease
- Inadequate surfactant production (as in premature infants)
- Pulmonary embolism

CLINICAL FEATURES

Medical History

Chief Complaints

Dependent on the severity of the atelectasis and the general health status of the patient. Severe atelectasis causes the patient to complain of difficult breathing. Fever may or may not be present.

History of Present Illness

Atelectasis most often occurs in patients with a recent history of abdominal or thoracic surgery.

Past Medical History

A history of chest cage deformities, such as kyphoscoliosis or neuromuscular disease, increases the risk of atelectasis.

Family History

Noncontributory.

Physical Examination

The findings on physical examination vary and depend on the amount of the lung involved with the atelectasis and the underlying condition of the lungs in general.

Vital signs: Rapid and shallow breathing are usually present; tachycardia may be present if pain or hypoxemia is occurring.

HEENT: Noncontributory.

Neck: Noncontributory.

Chest: Fine late-inspiratory crackles are often present in the dependent regions. Decreased resonance to percussion over the atelectatic region is common. Bronchial breath sounds may be heard if the larger airways are patent, leading into the area of atelectasis.

Abdomen: Noncontributory.

Extremities: Noncontributory.

Laboratory Data

ABG: Often demonstrates mild to moderate hypoxemia on room air with mild respiratory alkalosis.

Pulmonary function testing: Bedside spirometry demonstrates reduced vital capacity in most cases.

CBC: Often normal but may show elevated WBC count if pneumonia is also present.

Chest radiograph: One or more areas of increased white out; evidence of volume loss (e.g., elevated diaphragm) may be present if the atelectasis is severe.

TREATMENT

Treatment varies from case to case; the ideal treatment is to use lung expansion therapies (e.g., incentive spirometry) in high-risk patients (upper abdominal surgery patients) immediately after the surgery.

Patients with evidence of excessive airway secretions should have bronchial hygiene therapy before surgery and as part of the postoperative treatment plan.

IPPB or CPAP may be needed in patients unable to perform incentive spirometry because of a decreased level of consciousness.

Figure 4–1 outlines the treatment of atelectasis.

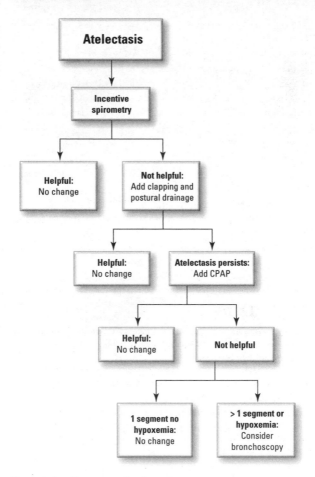

Figure 4–1. *Treatment of atelectasis.*

QUESTIONS FREQUENTLY ASKED BY PATIENT OR CAREGIVER

1. How often should I perform the incentive spirometry?

At least every 2 hours while awake and for 8 to 10 breaths each session.

2. Why do I sometimes get lightheaded when I use the incentive spirometer?

You are hyperventilating. You need to slow down and take pauses between each deep breath.

3. Why do I have to do the incentive spirometry?

Your doctor wants to make sure that your lungs remain well expanded. If you had surgery with general anesthesia, you may have a tendency to take small breaths and not keep your lungs fully expanded. Mucus can collect in the distal airways and this, along with shallow breathing, can lead to more serious lung problems like pneumonia.

4. How many days will I need to do the incentive spirometry?

It varies from patient to patient. Usually your doctor will discontinue the incentive spirometry after you are ambulating and the pain from the surgery has diminished.

5. Why has my doctor ordered this postural drainage with clapping on my chest?

This procedure helps move excessive mucus that is collecting in your lung toward your upper airway, where it can be more easily coughed out. Secretions that plug up distal airways can cause pneumonia and other lung problems.

6. I had surgery on my foot last year, and the doctor did not order incentive spirometry. Why has it been ordered this time for my gallbladder surgery?

The closer the surgical incision site is to the diaphragm, the more likely the surgery will lead to lung problems.

7. What can I do to help with the pain I feel over the abdominal incision site during deep breathing and coughing?

Use a firm pillow to act as an external splint. Also ask your nurse for pain medication when needed.

8. Should I cough even though it hurts?

Yes, but don't force it. A deep breath before a cough is good for expanding your lungs, and the coughing helps remove excessive lung mucus.

9. Many years ago, I had abdominal surgery and was given positive-pressure breathing treatments. Why are you not giving me those treatments this time?

Those were called "IPPB" treatments. Research has shown that incentive spirometry is just as effective and is associated with fewer complications and lower cost.

Reference

Wilkins, RL, and Dexter, JR: Respiratory Disease: A Case Study Approach to Patient Care, second edition. FA Davis, Philadelphia, 1998.

Chapter 5

Bronchiectasis

Bronchiectasis is a chronic and permanent dilatation of the bronchi caused by destruction of the elastic and muscular components of the bronchial walls. It may occur in an isolated area of the lung or in multiple sites.

KEY TERMS

bronchogram a radiologic examination in which the bronchi are outlined by a radio-opaque substance; once the gold standard for diagnosing bronchiectasis, it has been replaced by the CT scan

cylindric bronchiectasis–a pathologic type of bronchiectasis in which the affected bronchi do not taper off in diameter but rather come to an abrupt, squared end

fetid sputum–foul-smelling sputum

mucopurulent–a description of sputum that contains mucus and pus

saccular (cystic) bronchiectasis–severe form of bronchiectasis that results in ballooning of peripheral bronchi

EPIDEMIOLOGY

Unknown.

ETIOLOGY

Most often bronchiectasis occurs secondary to a lung infection. Pertussis and infections associated with cystic fibrosis are the two most common causes of bronchiectasis.

CLINICAL FEATURES

Medical History

Chief Complaints

Chronic cough producing foul-smelling sputum. Dyspnea may also be present if the disease is severe or if an underlying diffuse lung disease (e.g., CF) is also present.

History of Present Illness

Patients often present with a chronic cough that produces a large volume of foul-smelling sputum.

Past Medical History

Usually the patient has had frequent lung infections.

Physical Examination

HEENT: Often normal.

Neck: Noncontributory.

Chest: Localized area of coarse crackles; expiratory rhonchi are a common finding; decreased resonance to percussion may be heard over areas of consolidation.

Extremities: Digital clubbing may be present but is not common.

Laboratory Data

CBC: May be normal or demonstrate increased WBC count with infection.

Chest radiograph: May be normal if the bronchiectasis is mild and localized. In most cases, tubular shadows are seen as paired parallel or slightly tapered line shadows extending distally and following a bronchovascular distribution. Atelectasis may be seen in more severe cases. Loss of lung volume is sometimes present in some areas, and hyperinflation may be seen in other areas.

Bronchography may be used to demonstrate the bronchiectasis, but CT scans are now the favored way to establish a definitive diagnosis.

ABG: Typically demonstrates nonspecific changes such as hypoxemia on room air. Elevation of CO_2 may occur if advanced disease is present.

PFT: Often demonstrates decreased expiratory flow measurements, especially in advanced cases.

Bronchiectasis

TREATMENT

The goal of treatment is to control the patient's symptoms and prevent progression of the disease. The basics of treatment are:

- Antibiotics are often needed and are prescribed according to results of sputum culture and sensitivity results.
- Bronchial hygiene is often a major component of treatment, especially in cases in which the patient is producing excessive amounts of sputum.

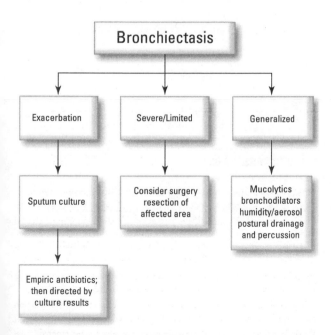

Figure 5–1. *Treatment of bronchiectasis.*

Pocket Guide to Respiratory Disease | **35**

- Humidity and aerosol therapy are needed to thin secretions and assist with their removal.
- Bronchodilators are often useful for reversing bronchospasm.
- Surgical resection of the bronchiectic region is possible but is reserved for specific cases when the patient is young and able to tolerate the procedure and the disease is interfering with daily life functions. Surgical resection is also done when major hemorrhage from a bronchiectic region is present.

Figure 5–1 outlines the treatment of bronchiectasis.

QUESTIONS FREQUENTLY ASKED BY PATIENT OR CAREGIVER

1. I can't stop coughing. What can be done?

People with bronchiectasis always cough and produce sputum. The goal of the treatment is to minimize the sputum production and make it easier to cough out. Your coughing should decrease when the disorder is more stable with treatment but probably will not go away completely.

2. Why do I have bronchiectasis? What did I do to cause this?

Bronchiectasis develops after infection damages the walls of one or more airways in the lung. In the past, whooping cough was the most common cause of bronchiectasis but because the pertussis vaccine has been commonly used, bronchiectasis is becoming much less common. Other lung diseases such as TB and CF that cause chronic airway injury can cause bronchiectasis. You did not do anything to cause this disorder. You were just unlucky to have an illness that damaged your airways.

3. What kind of damage is done and how does the infection cause the airway damage?

Chronic infection in the airway causes scarring around the outside of one or more airway walls. This scarring is responsible for traction that pulls the airway open in a specific segment. Air flowing through this area slows down because of the localized widening of the airway walls and sputum tends to collect in the defective regions. The slow-flowing air cannot push sputum upward toward the trachea for clearance, even with good coughing. This collection of sputum is an excellent medium that favors growth of bacteria, which causes more injury to the airway wall.

4. What treatments are available?

Numerous treatments are available. If the bronchiectasis is severe but limited to a single segment or lobe, it can be surgically removed (assuming that lung function is good enough to tolerate the procedure). Antibiotics do not cure the disease but are important in reducing symptoms and minimizing future damage. Mucolytics thin the sputum and make it easier to cough out, which is important. In addition, postural drainage and clapping also help mobilize secretions stuck in the airways.

5. What germs cause the infections in my lungs, and why do I always get the same antibiotics?

Pseudomonas and often gram-negative rods are the most common organisms causing infection in people with bronchiectasis. The antibiotics your physician has ordered are specifically designed to destroy these organisms.

6. Are there any new treatments for bronchiectasis?

Yes, a new form of tobramycin called TOBI is now available in a form that can be inhaled from a small-volume nebulizer. Previous forms of the drug were available only as an IV treatment, which required home health IV therapy or hospitalization. Pulmozyme is a genetically engineered enzyme that breaks down the protein in sputum and makes it easier to cough up. It has been shown to help people with CF and may help patients with bronchiectasis.

7. Of all these treatments we have talked about, which ones should I be taking?

I know a lot about the treatments available for bronchiectasis, but I don't know as much about your specific case. Specific recommendations for treatment should only be made by your doctor after a history and physical examination and review of your records.

8. I cough up lots of green sputum every day. Does that mean I should always be taking antibiotics?

Your doctor will have the final say on this, but antibiotics are typically used when your sputum becomes darker in color or increases in quantity. Bronchiectasis is one of the few diseases in which long-term use of antibiotics may be helpful if sputum is constantly produced in large amounts and is dark in color.

9. Are the germs in my sputum contagious?

Almost certainly not. Most of the germs causing infection in your airways are commonly found in water and in the mouths of most people. They are a problem only to people with injured lungs or those with compromised immune systems. You can be around elderly people and infants unless you have been found to have TB.

10. Why do you keep giving me breathing treatments?

Bronchiectasis is not usually helped by bronchodilator treatments, but many people with bronchiectasis also have some bronchospasm (asthma) that does respond favorably to bronchodilator treatments. The humidity/aerosol treatments are also helpful in mobilizing thick mucus in the lung.

Reference

Wilkins, RL, and Dexter, JR: Respiratory Disease: A Case Study Approach to Patient Care, second edition. FA Davis, Philadelphia, 1998.

Chapter 6

Bronchopulmonary Dysplasia

BPD is a chronic lung disease seen in infants who required mechanical ventilation because of RDS. The hallmarks are pulmonary fibrosis and bronchiolar metaplasia with V/Q mismatching.

KEY TERMS

barotrauma–trauma to the lungs caused by the use of positive pressure ventilation (PPV)

metaplasia–the changing of normal cells to abnormal cells because of chronic injury

PDA–failure of the ductus arteriosus to close after birth

volutrauma–trauma to the lungs because of excessive expansion with large mechanical tidal volumes

EPIDEMIOLOGY

Incidence varies because of the lack of a standardized definition. Related inversely to the patient's gestational age and weight.

ETIOLOGY

More common in white males, prematurity, oxygen therapy, mechanical ventilation (especially with high pressures), barotrauma, volutrauma, vitamin deficiency, PDA, fluid overload, perinatal asphyxia, infection (CMV, chlamydia, ureaplasma), family history of asthma.

CLINICAL FEATURES

Medical History

Chief Complaints

Difficulty weaning from mechanical ventilation, pulmonary edema, sensitivity to changes in FIO_2.

History of Present Illness

Presence of one or several of the etiologic factors.

Past Medical History

Prematurity with low birth weight.

Family History

History of asthma or previous sibling with BPD may be present.

Occupational and Social History

Noncontributory.

Physical Examination

General appearance is respiratory distress and increased work of breathing. Oxygen therapy in use.

Vital Signs: Tachycardia and tachypnea.

Sensorium: Normal.

HEENT: Audible grunting, nasal flaring.

Neck: Normal.

Chest:

Inspection: Subcostal and intercostal retractions.

Auscultation: Diffuse fine crackles and wheezes.

Abdomen: Normal.

Extremities: Normal.

Laboratory Data

ABG: Compensated or partially compensated respiratory acidosis with hypoxemia.

PFT: Increased airway resistance.

Chest radiograph: Areas of irregular densities (atelectasis) with areas of hyperlucency (hyperinflation).

Other data: Rule out pneumonia, PDA, sepsis, and IVH.

TREATMENT

Supportive: Adequate nutrition and oxygenation. Mechanical ventilation with low PIPs, bronchodilators, diuretics, steroids, and careful fluid management.

QUESTIONS FREQUENTLY ASKED BY PATIENT OR CAREGIVER

1. Why did my child get this disease?

Your child got this disease because of injury to his or her lung. Prematurity and mechanical ventilation predispose infants to this type of injury.

2. Is it hereditary?

BPD is not hereditary. However, there is a familial tendency that is related to the severity of RDS and thus the risk of BPD. If a family has a preterm infant who has severe RDS, a subsequent preterm infant who has RDS would likely also have severe disease and be at increased risk for BPD.

3. Will it get any better?

In most infants with BPD, as the lung continues to grow, its function should improve.

4. Is it fatal or life threatening?

BPD is usually not life threatening; however, there are a small number of infants who have such severe lung disease that they will die. You should discuss your child's case with the attending physician for a more specific prognosis in this case.

5. Are the lungs permanently damaged?

Most infants with BPD will lead normal lives. However, there are usually abnormalities of lung function that will be present for the infant's lifetime.

6. What are the other complications of this disease?

Many infants with BPD have problems with reactive airway disease (asthma). Also, they have an increased risk of infection, particularly during the first 2 years of life.

7. What kind of home care will it require?

The majority of infants with BPD do not have special home care needs. However, some of these infants may need supplemental oxygen for several weeks to months. They may also require inhaled medications. In a very few cases, some infants require prolonged mechanical ventilation for months to years. Also, some infants require prolonged use of certain medications.

8. Can the child lead a normal life?

Yes. Most children with BPD lead normal lives. Some with severe disease may spontaneously choose a more sedentary life.

9. Will my child be oxygen dependent?

Most infants with BPD are successfully weaned from supplemental oxygen before they go home; however, some infants may require supplemental oxygen for several months after discharge from the NICU.

10. Are there long-term side effects from medication?

It is unlikely that children with BPD who require long-term medications will have any side effects. The most common long-term medications that are used for infants with BPD are inhaled medications that dilate the airways and inhaled medications that decrease the inflammation of the airways. These are the same types of drugs that are used for children who have chronic asthma.

Chapter 7

Chest Trauma

Chest trauma is a serious problem because of the nature of the organs enclosed in the chest and their importance in maintaining life. A large variety of abnormalities may occur in patients who have experienced blunt chest trauma.

KEY TERMS

aortic rupture–a sudden tear of the aorta caused by blunt chest trauma

bronchopleural fistula–an abnormal opening between the lung and the pleura that leads to a continuous leak of air into the pleural space

cardiac contusion–bruising of the heart caused by blunt chest trauma

cardiac tamponade–compression of the heart caused by a buildup of blood in the pericardium

flail chest–a condition that occurs when two or more ribs are broken in more than one place, resulting in a section of the chest wall's moving (flailing) independently from the rest of the chest wall

hemothorax–blood in the pleural space

lung contusion–an injury to the lung as the result of blunt trauma to the chest, causing pathologic changes in the lung similar to a bruise

pneumothorax–air in the pleural space

subcutaneous emphysema–air in the subcutaneous tissues caused by leaking from the lung

EPIDEMIOLOGY

Trauma is responsible for more than 130,000 deaths and 70 million injuries in the US each year. It is the leading cause of death among people under the age of 40 years. The most common causes of trauma are motor vehicle accidents, accidental falls, gunshot wounds, and stab wounds. About 25% of all trauma deaths are caused by injuries to the chest.

ETIOLOGY

Not applicable.

CLINICAL FEATURES

The clinical features vary widely with the severity of the trauma and the underlying health status of the patient.

Medical History

Chief Complaints

Pain, dyspnea, and shock are common.

History of Present Illness

Should describe the nature of the accident and the location on the body of the injuries. The possibility of neck injury should be noted in addition to the chest trauma.

Past Medical History

Not applicable.

Physical Examination

This is an important part of the assessment because it describes the location and nature of the injuries to the chest.

HEENT: Pupils should be inspected for their response to light in the comatose patient. The neck should be inspected for evidence of trauma. The position of the trachea should be noted because it could shift to one side if the mediastinum is displaced to one side.

Chest: Evidence of bruising, flail chest, subcutaneous emphysema, and open chest wound should be noted. Percussion should be done to assess for pneumothorax (increased resonance) or hemothorax (decreased resonance). Fractured ribs often cause pain and guarded and shallow breathing.

Heart sounds will be diminished when cardiac tamponade is present.

Abdomen: May be distended if bleeding has occurred into the abdomen.

Extremities: Should be inspected for evidence of trauma, color, and temperature.

Clinical Laboratory Data

Anemia may be present if bleeding has been extensive. Leukocytosis is often present in response to the trauma.

Electrolytes are usually normal.

Chest radiograph: May show pulmonary contusion, pneumothorax, fractured ribs, and widening of the mediastinum if bleeding in the chest is present.

ABG: Usually demonstrates hypoxemia with or without respiratory acidosis.

TREATMENT

Goals of respiratory care treatment are to:

- Obtain and maintain an airway; intubation is recommended in most cases; be sure the tube is in good position by listening for breath sounds and using portable chest radiograph.
- Provide adequate oxygenation and ventilation; usually a high FIO_2 and mechanical ventilation are needed to maintain adequate gas exchange when severe chest trauma has occurred.
- Provide humidity and aerosol therapy as needed to assist with secretion removal and reverse bronchospasm, if present.
- Chest tubes may need to be placed if pneumothorax or hemothorax are present.
- Hemodynamic monitoring is important to maintain appropriate fluid levels and cardiac output.
- PEEP therapy is often needed when refractory hypoxemia is a problem. This may occur 48 to 72 hours after the original injuries.
- Medication to control pain is an important part of the overall treatment plan.

QUESTIONS FREQUENTLY ASKED BY PATIENT OR CAREGIVER

1. The doctor says I have a pneumothorax. What is that? Will my lung be permanently damaged?

This is caused by air leaking out of the lung and into a space between the rib cage and the lung. A small pneumothorax may not need treatment, but larger ones require a chest tube to drain out the air. In either case, the lung will return to normal function.

---

2. I hit the steering wheel hard but did not break any ribs or bones. Why am I having so much trouble breathing?

The lung can become bruised, just like your arms or legs. A sudden blow to the chest will bruise the lung and make it function less effectively for a week or two. It should slowly resolve and return to normal function.

---

3. How long will I have to have this chest tube in my side?

Doctors leave chest tubes in place until there has been no air leak for a day or more and less than 2 to 3 oz of fluid drains out per day.

---

4. Why did they put my husband on a ventilator after the car accident? His rib cage was broken, but the doctor said his lungs were not damaged by the accident. Why did they not just fix the ribs like they fixed his broken leg?

Your husband's chest wall must be stable for the lungs to work effectively. When more than a few ribs are broken in two or more places, the chest wall is unstable and ventilation is difficult. Doctors have tried wiring the ribs together, but that never worked well. Using the ventilator as an "internal splint" makes the broken ribs move in synchrony with the unbroken ribs and allows better healing of the broken ribs.

5. The doctor says I have a hemothorax. What is that and how is it treated?

Hemothorax is when blood leaks from the lung into the space between the lung and the chest wall. It is treated by insertion of a chest tube to drain out the fluid if the amount of blood in the lung is significant. After the bleeding stops and the tube is not draining blood any more, the tube can be removed and your lung should return to normal.

6. (Patient writes question on bedside chalkboard.) How long will I have to have this tube in my throat and be on the ventilator?

This is difficult to predict and is determined by how quickly your lungs heal and how quickly you are able to breathe on your own. It would be best to ask your physician for more exact details.

7. I heard one of the doctors say I have a cardiac tamponade. What is that, and is it serious?

This occurs when blood accumulates in the sac around the heart. It can be serious and can lead to poor cardiac function. Your doctor has implemented good treatment and we expect the problem to resolve completely.

8. (This question is from a family member of a patient with head trauma and a suspected neck injury after arrival to the ICU from the emergency room.) My brother looks so uncomfortable with the breathing tube going through his nose. Isn't it better to have the breathing tube go through his mouth?

Usually the breathing tubes are put into the mouth, but placing an endotracheal tube through the mouth requires the doctor to move the patient's neck. If there is a question about a neck injury and the patient requires intubation, then the tube is usually placed through the nose or surgically through the skin of the neck.

9. What is a myocardial contusion?

A myocardial contusion is an injury to the heart. This is usually the result of a severe chest injury, usually in the breastbone area. Immediately after a significant injury, a myocardial contusion can cause heart arrhythmias, some of which can be serious. It also causes chest pain, ECG changes that look like a heart attack, and disruption of the normal electrical pathways in the heart. Sometimes patients who develop a myocardial contusion must be watched in the ICU, but most improve as the injury heals.

10. My daughter hit her head when she had a motorcycle accident. The doctors say that the ventilator is breathing for my daughter to reduce the pressure in her head. What do they mean?

One problem that develops from a brain injury is swelling of the injured areas of the brain. The brain is surrounded by bone, so even a small amount of swelling could make the situation much worse. Breathing for her, especially hyperventilation, causes a reduction of swelling in the injured areas of the brain and reduces the potential for additional brain damage.

Reference

Wilkins, RL, and Dexter, JR: Respiratory Disease: A Case Study Approach to Patient Care, second edition. FA Davis, Philadelphia, 1998.

Chapter 8

Chronic Bronchitis

Chronic bronchitis is an obstructive lung disease characterized by a persistent productive cough for at least 3 months of the year for at least 2 consecutive years. It is a common problem among smokers and leads to a progressive decrease in airflow.

KEY TERMS

COPD—a disease state characterized by the presence of airflow obstruction that is usually progressive and caused by chronic bronchitis, emphysema, or both

cor pulmonale—right heart failure caused by chronic hypoxemic lung disease

phlegm—mucus from the tracheobronchial tree not contaminated by oral secretions

sputum—secretions from the lung that have been expelled by coughing

EPIDEMIOLOGY

- Chronic bronchitis is a problem around the world, especially in countries where cigarette smoking is common.
- Approximately 14 million Americans have COPD and 12.5 million of those with COPD have predominantly chronic bronchitis.
- Approximately 4% to 6% of men and 1% to 3% of women in the U.S. have COPD.
- COPD is the fourth most common cause of death in the U.S.

ETIOLOGY

- Cigarette smoking is the most common factor associated with the onset of chronic bronchitis.

- Heavy exposure to smog, occupational dusts and fumes, low birth weight, genetics, and gender may play roles in the disease but are probably distant issues compared with cigarette use.

CLINICAL FEATURES

Medical History

Chief Complaints

Episodic dyspnea, cough, and sputum production are most common; fever may occur with infection.

History of Present Illness

Patients have chronic cough with sputum production that worsens during episodes of infection. Dyspnea occurs only during the episodes of infection early in the disease, but occurs with minimal exertion in advanced cases.

Past Medical History

Significant smoking history.

Family History

May be positive for chronic lung disease.

Occupational and Social History

Not applicable.

Physical Examination

Vital signs: May be stable at rest; fever present with infection; tachycardia and tachypnea may be present when acute hypoxemia occurs during bouts with infection.

Neck: Jugular venous distension often present; use of accessory muscles may be seen.

Chest: Right ventricular heave present at sternal border; expiratory wheezes and rhonchi heard during auscultation; prolonged expiratory phase.

Abdomen: Hepatomegaly commonly palpated.

Extremities: Pedal edema common; cyanosis may be seen.

Laboratory Data

ABG: Compensated respiratory acidosis with hypoxemia common; acute respiratory acidosis (elevated $PaCO_2$ and low pH) indicates acute ventilatory failure.

CBC: Elevated RBC count, hemoglobin and hematocrit are often seen; WBC may be elevated with infection.

PFT: Reduced expiratory flow rates; normal vital capacity and TLC.

Chest radiograph: Often normal in mild to moderate cases; may show hyperinflation with acute episodes of airway infection.

Sputum gram stain: Numerous pus cells when bacterial infection is present.

TREATMENT

- Correct hypoxemia if $PaO_2 < 55$ mm Hg or if the PaO_2 is 55 to 60 mm Hg and evidence of cor pulmonale is present; low-flow oxygen therapy usually effective; goal is to obtain a PaO_2 of 60 to 80 mm Hg or SaO_2 of 90% to 92%.
- Recognize and treat any acute problems such as infection, heart failure, or bronchospasm.
- Treat airway obstruction with bronchodilators:
  - Provide a fast-acting bronchodilator (e.g., albuterol or ipratropium bromide) as a rescue drug when acute dyspnea occurs; add the other bronchodilator for persistent dyspnea.
  - Provide a long-acting bronchodilator (ipratropium bromide, salmeterol, or both) for long-term relief of bronchospasm.
  - Add steroid (e.g., prednisone) if the above does not provide relief during an acute episode of dyspnea caused by bronchospasm.
- Provide humidity and aerosol therapy when evidence of retained secretions is present (e.g., loose, nonproductive cough; atelectasis on chest radiograph)
- Encourage the patient to attend smoking cessation program by pointing out the benefits to the lungs.
- Evaluate the patient for potential benefit of pulmonary rehabilitation program.

Figure 8–1 outlines the treatment of COPD.

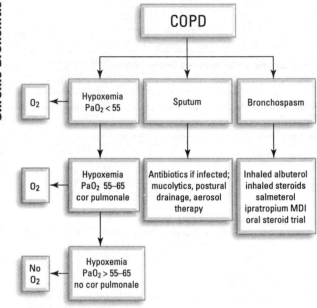

Figure 8–1. *Treatment of COPD.*

QUESTIONS FREQUENTLY ASKED BY PATIENT OR CAREGIVER

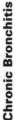

1. Why do I cough up so much sputum?

The major problem with chronic bronchitis is hypertrophy (enlargement) and hyperplasia (increased number) of the mucus glands. This results in large amounts of sputum production into your airways, which is eventually coughed out.

2. When should I take antibiotics?

Always consult with your physician first. He or she will usually want to hear from you if your sputum increases in amount or changes color.

3. Can I become addicted to the oxygen?

No, oxygen is not addictive. Its value is primarily in preventing pulmonary hypertension and right heart failure, which reduces hospital visits and increased life expectancy. Be sure to use it only as your doctor prescribes.

4. Can I become addicted to the bronchodilators or steroids?

No, but bronchodilators such as Ventolin become less effective with use over time, so higher doses may be needed. Steroids can cause a decrease in adrenal function so that abrupt discontinuing may cause problems such as fatigue and hypotension.

5. What are the side effects of the steroids?

Use of oral steroids may lead to cataracts; diabetes; osteoporosis; round face; weight gain; and thin, bruising skin. The inhaled steroids are not associated with these types of systemic side effects but may lead to oral thrush.

6. Why do my ankles swell?

Chronic lung disease can lead to ankle swelling because the lack of oxygen in the lung causes the pulmonary blood vessels to constrict and may result in the right side of the heart working extra hard to pump blood through the lung. As a result, the heart may fail to pump blood adequately and a backup of blood into the lower extremities can cause ankle swelling. The treatment your doctor has prescribed should help eliminate this problem. If it does not improve over the next month, let your doctor know.

7. Why is a spacer needed for the pocket inhaler?

The spacer makes it easier for you to inhale the medication and helps make coordination of squeezing the MDI and inhaling less critical. It also results in less medication landing in your mouth, where it is not needed and side effects are more common, and more medication ending up in the lung where it is needed.

8. Is it too late to stop smoking?

No! When you stop smoking, the rapid decline in lung function associated with cigarette use is reduced significantly. This is always helpful.

9. Sometimes there is blood in my sputum. Does this mean I have lung cancer?

Probably not, because bronchitis is a common cause of bloody sputum. You should mention this to your physician so that he or she can rule out other possible causes.

10. Do you know of any support groups for people with COPD like myself?

You can contact the local chapter of the American Lung Association by looking in your phone book or calling Information.

11. Is there any medicine that will get rid of all this sputum?

No, the sputum is coming from your airways, and we cannot stop the sputum production. Drinking plenty of water will help make it easier to cough up the sputum. Some medications may make it easier to expectorate the sputum. Ask your doctor about this.

Reference

Wilkins, RL, and Dexter, JR: Respiratory Disease: A Case Study Approach to Patient Care, second edition. FA Davis, Philadelphia, 1998.

Chapter 9

Croup

Croup is also known as laryngotracheal bronchitis. It is caused by a viral infection of the larynx, trachea, and bronchi. In most cases, it is mild and responds well to treatment. Occasionally, a patient with a more severe episode who does not respond to initial treatment may need to be hospitalized. (Although the chapter in the accompanying textbook, *Respiratory Disease: A Case Study Approach to Patient Care*, 2nd edition, addresses epiglottitis as well as croup, the authors have decided to focus strictly on croup in this chapter because the recent development of a vaccine for epiglottitis and the subsequent decline in its incidence.)

KEY TERMS

epiglottitis–bacterial infection of the epiglottis, aryepiglottic folds, and aretynoids

lymphadenopathy–swelling of the lymph glands

racemic epinephrine–a beta-adrenergic medication given to a patient with croup by aerosol to shrink swollen mucous membranes and relieve dyspnea

steeple sign–a term for the narrow, pointed appearance of the subglottic area on radiography; it is caused by tissue inflammation and swelling

stridor–the high-pitched monophonic wheeze heard during inspiration and sometimes expiration caused by the narrowing of the upper airway

EPIDEMIOLOGY

Most often found in children aged 6 months to 3 years; more common in males.

ETIOLOGY

Viral in origin; caused by parainfluenza, influenza, RSV, adenovirus; more common in winter.

CLINICAL FEATURES

Medical History

Chief Complaints

Slow onset of respiratory distress, fever, cough, runny nose.

History of Present Illness

Fever for 1 to 2 days, nasal congestion, and coughing with a distinctive barking quality that seems worse at night.

Past Medical History

Noncontributory.

Family History

Noncontributory.

Occupational and Social History

Noncontributory.

Physical Examination

General appearance may be anxious, in obvious respiratory distress.

Vital Signs: Tachycardia, tachypnea, mild fever may be present.

Sensorium: Normal; diminished could indicate respiratory failure.

HEENT: Nasal flaring, dried nasal mucus, red throat.

Neck: Normal or mild lymphadenopathy.

Chest:

Inspection: Retractions common with severe cases.

Palpation: Normal.

Percussion: Normal.

Auscultation: Inspiratory stridor is most common; inspiratory and expiratory stridor in severe cases.

Abdomen: Normal.

Extremities: Normal.

Laboratory Data

ABG: Mild hypoxemia, but usually not done.

PFT: Not indicated.

Chest radiography: "Steeple sign" (subglottic narrowing), possible infiltrates.

Other Data

CBC: Normal.

Culture and sensitivity of sputum: Normal.

TREATMENT

Cool mist, oxygen, racemic epinephrine.

Figure 9–1 compares the presentation and treatment of stridor in croup and epiglottitis.

QUESTIONS FREQUENTLY ASKED BY PATIENT OR CAREGIVER

1. What is croup?

Laryngotracheobronchitis or viral croup is the major cause of acute upper airway obstruction in children. It is an infection caused by a variety of viruses.

2. Why does my child make that noise when he or she breathes?

The virus infection is primarily localized to the larynx and trachea, and the resultant inflammation and swelling have caused your child's airway to be narrowed. The obstruction to airflow results in the inspiratory stridor and difficulty in breathing.

3. Why does my child look worse when he or she cries or is upset?

Being upset or worried decreases the child's ability to manage the airway obstruction. For this reason, it is important to keep your child calm and comfortable. It also increases the demand on the lungs to supply more ventilation and may make the obstruction seem worse.

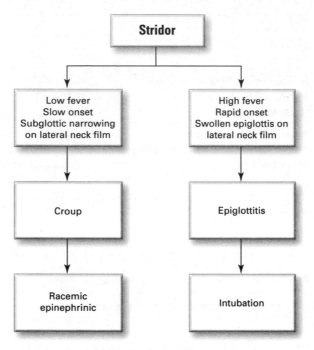

Figure 9–1. *Stridor in croup and epiglottitis.*

4. My child's grandmother says that warm mist will help his or her breathing. Can mist be used?

The benefits of mist therapy have not been demonstrated, so we no longer use it in hospitalized patients. In addition, it may increase your child's anxiety.

5. How long will this breathing difficulty last?

Symptoms usually last a total of 7 to 14 days. By the time medical attention is sought, symptoms usually last 4 more days.

6. Will my child get worse?

It's unlikely. Only a minority of hospitalized patients have symptoms that progress to severe. Among children hospitalized for croup, fewer than 1% require an artificial airway on a temporary basis.

7. What is the medication you are giving?

It is epinephrine or adrenaline. It decreases the swelling in the larynx and subglottic area, which makes it easier for your child to breathe.

8. Why do you have to give the epinephrine so often?

The effect of epinephrine is short-lived and it does not alter the natural history of the airway obstruction; therefore, your child's breathing becomes more difficult when the effect wears off.

9. Does epinephrine cause the disease to last longer?

No.

10. Why is my doctor prescribing corticosteroids for my child?

Many physicians prescribe steroids to suppress the inflammatory response and decrease the swelling in viral croup. Studies have demonstrated more rapid improvement when steroids are used in children with severe viral croup.

11. Will the steroids harm my child?

There is no evidence of any ill effects of a short course of steroids used in children with viral croup, but that is a good question to discuss with your doctor.

12. Why does my child need oxygen?

Hypoxemia usually indicates that the virus is also involving the lower airways, which interferes with oxygen exchange. It is temporary and will probably be discontinued in a day or two.

13. How will I know when to call my doctor or bring my child into the ER if this problem occurs again?

Signs of more severe illness are fever of greater than 101°F, severely labored breathing at rest, and noisy breathing on inspiration and exhalation.

References

Kaditis, AG, and Wald, ER. Viral croup: Current diagnosis and treatment. *Pediatr Infect Dis J* 1998, 17:827–834.

Klassen, TP. Recent advances in one treatment of bronchiolitis and laryngitis. *Pediatr Clin North Am* 1997, 44:249–261.

Wilkins, RL, and Dexter, JR: Respiratory Disease: A Case Study Approach to Patient Care, second edition. FA Davis, Philadelphia, 1998.

Chapter 10

Cystic Fibrosis

CF is a chronic obstructive lung disease that is the most common lethal genetic disease in Americans of European descent. It is most often diagnosed in childhood and affects numerous body systems in addition to the lungs.

KEY TERMS

autosomal recessive–a genetic trait controlled by two genes; a recessive trait will not be present unless both parents contribute one recessive gene

bronchiectasis–an abnormal dilatation of a bronchus or several bronchi in the lungs

dornase alfa (Pulmozyme)–a therapeutic agent used to thin thick mucus in the lungs

nasal polyps–an abnormal growth located in the nasal structures

sweat chloride test–a laboratory test done to assist diagnosing CF; an electrolyte concentration greater than 60 mEq/L in children is consistent with CF in children

tram tracks–parallel lines seen on the chest radiography caused by thickening of the bronchial walls in patients with CF

EPIDEMIOLOGY

The odds of any white adult being a carrier of the CF gene are somewhere between one in 16 to one in 25. The incidence is much lower in other races.

Approximately one baby in 2500 births of white children in the U.S. has CF. The incidence is about one in 17,000 for African-American babies.

ETIOLOGY

CF is an inherited autosomal recessive disease. This means that one CF gene is donated from each parent to the child so that the child has two genes for CF. Children with CF inherit the disease when they get one abnormal CF gene from each parent.

CLINICAL FEATURES

Medical History

Chief Complaints

Patients with CF often complain of cough, sputum production, and dyspnea. Fever and wheezing are other common symptoms.

History of Present Illness

The patient often complains of a recent increase in sputum, fever, and cough caused by the onset of a respiratory infection. Hemoptysis is often seen in more advanced cases.

Past Medical History

Frequent episodes of respiratory infections and lack of weight gain.

Family History

Child may have a brother or sister with CF.

Occupational and Social History

Not applicable.

Physical Examination

HEENT: Nasal polyps are common.

Neck: JVD may be seen in more advanced cases when cor pulmonale is present. Use of accessory muscles is common in more advanced cases or when acute obstruction is present.

Chest: Coarse crackles and expiratory wheezing are frequently heard. Breathing is often labored. Evidence of hyperinflation (barrel chest) is often seen.

Abdomen: Patient often appears malnourished.

Extremities: Clubbing may be seen in advanced cases.

Laboratory Data

Sweat chloride levels: >60 mEq/L in children; >80 mEq/L in adults.

PFT: Reduced expiratory flows; increased residual volume and reduced FVC in advanced cases.

ABG: Mild to moderate hypoxemia; respiratory acidosis in advanced cases.

Chest radiography: Evidence of hyperinflation as seen by low, flat diaphragm and a large retrosternal airspace; tram tracks are often present. The radiograph should be checked for evidence of pneumothorax, atelectasis, and pneumonia.

TREATMENT

Selected vitamins are given as a nutritional supplement. Respiratory care provides humidity and aerosol therapy to assist the patient in clearing retained pulmonary secretions. Postural drainage and clapping are also done for similar reasons. Bronchodilators are given by aerosol to reduce wheezing and shortness of breath. Antibiotics are frequently needed to overcome lung infections. Mucolytic agents are useful when secretions are thick and difficult to expectorate. Inhaled dornase alfa (Pulmozyme) is almost always given to patients with CF to help thin the thick secretions. Most patients with CF also receive inhaled tobramycin (TOBI) twice a day every other month. The use of inhaled dornase alfa may prove useful for secretion removal, although the cost is prohibitive.

The treatment for cystic fibrosis is similar to that for bronchiectasis, outlined in Figure 10–1.

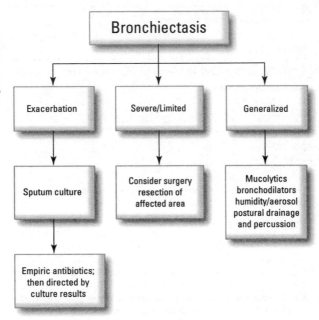

Figure 10–1. *Treatment of bronchiectasis.*

QUESTIONS FREQUENTLY ASKED BY PATIENT OR CAREGIVER

I. How long can I expect my child with CF to live?

New advances in the treatment of patients with CF help them to live much longer than in the past and to have a better quality of life. It is currently common for CF patients to live well into their 30s.

2. Is there a cure for this disease?

No, but research for a cure is currently under way and is progressing rapidly.

3. What are the odds of our having another child with CF?

The odds are one in four.

4. When should I contact the doctor if my child gets sick?

Whenever you sense that your child has developed new or more severe symptoms, you should contact the doctor. Look especially for evidence of infection, such as fever, increased sputum production, or a change in the color or character of the sputum. Report evidence of difficult breathing.

5. Why does my child not gain weight?

Pancreatic function is impaired and results in poor digestion and absorption of food. Patients with CF also have a higher than normal metabolic rate at rest.

6. Should I restrict my child's participation in exercise and sports?

No. Encourage exercise, at least to the point where your child can tolerate it, but do not allow extreme exertion that causes severe shortness of breath. Have your child avoid heavy exercise during hot days because this causes excessive loss of salt through sweat.

7. Why is the sputum produced so thick?

Recurrent respiratory infections are frequently associated with thick sputum. Encourage your child to drink lots of water.

8. Why are clapping and postural drainage helpful?

This procedure helps mobilize mucus from deep in the lung toward the upper airway, where it can be coughed out easier. If secretions are not coughed out, they can plug up the patient's bronchial tubes. This causes long-term damage to the lungs.

9. What new treatments are available?

Dornase alfa (Pulmozyme) to thin secretions is now available and has proven helpful. Inhaled TOBI provides much higher antibiotic levels than previous versions of tobramycin. Gene therapy has been tried but has shown only limited success. Other new drugs are being tested currently to help thin mucus and improve lung function.

10. Why is my child's kiss so salty?

The basic CF defect is a gene malfunction that produces a cell wall protein. This does not help cells to move salt well. Therefore, your child's skin and secretions contain more salt than those of most children. This same defect results in thick secretions. Thick sputum is hard to cough up and contributes to frequent lung infections.

11. If a patient with CF gets a lung transplant, does the disease attack the new lung?

No. The donor's lungs do not have the CF gene and will not develop CF.

12. My doctor says I have another infection with *Pseudomonas* organisms. This is the third infection by this bug this year. Why do I keep getting infections from this organism?

We are not sure why, but patients with CF are prone to infections caused by *Pseudomonas* organisms. The combination of excessive secretions in the airways and lungs and stagnation of these secretions contribute to the onset of infection in those with CF. This is why it is very important that you continue with your bronchial hygiene therapy very consistently.

Reference

Wilkins, RL, and Dexter, JR: Respiratory Disease: A Case Study Approach to Patient Care, second edition. FA Davis, Philadelphia, 1998.

Chapter 11

Emphysema

Emphysema is a COPD associated with abnormal dilatation of the distal air spaces. In patients with panlobular emphysema, all the airways distal to the terminal bronchioles are involved. In those with centrilobular emphysema, the distal air spaces are spared and only the more central airways are abnormal.

KEY TERMS

abdominal paradox–an abnormal breathing pattern associated with diaphragm fatigue in which the abdomen sinks inward with each inspiratory effort

alpha$_1$-antitrypsin–a plasma protein that inhibits the enzyme trypsin. Also known as an alpha protease inhibitor; a deficiency of this protein causes a hereditary form of panacinar emphysema

barrel chest–an abnormal increase in the A-P diameter of the chest caused by hyperinflation of the lung; most often caused by emphysema

bullectomy–surgical removal of one or more large bullae

bulla–a large collection of air within the lung caused by destruction of lung tissue with air trapping

Hoover's sign–an abnormal breathing pattern seen in patients with severe emphysema, in which the lateral portions of the lower chest wall move inward with each inspiratory effort

pneumoplasty–a surgical procedure performed on patients with severe emphysema to remove overdistended and functionless lung tissue; also know as lung volume reduction surgery

EPIDEMIOLOGY

Emphysema is a worldwide problem, especially in countries where cigarette smoking is common. Approximately 14 million Americans have COPD, and many of these people also suffer from some degree of emphysema. The number of Americans with emphysema as the predominant part of the COPD is approximately 2 million.

ETIOLOGY

Cigarette smoking is the most common factor associated with the onset of emphysema. Alpha$_1$-antitrypsin deficiency accounts for a small percentage (1%) of the patients with emphysema.

CLINICAL FEATURES

Medical History

Chief Complaints

Progressive dyspnea with exertion; dyspnea at rest occurs with more severe cases.

History of Present Illness

Patient reports a gradual increase in dyspnea with exertion. Initially the shortness of breath occurs only with significant exertion (e.g., walking up a flight of stairs), but it eventually begins to occur with minimal exertion. Exacerbation occurs with viral infections of the airways or lungs. Patients often note significant weight loss over the past several years because of a decrease in appetite.

Past Medical History

Significant smoking history.

Family History

Often positive for chronic lung disease.

Occupational and Social History

May be significant if patient is exposed to dust or fumes at work and smokes cigarettes.

Physical Examination

Vital signs: May be normal at rest or show minimal tachycardia and tachypnea. Pursed-lip breathing is often seen.

Neck: Significant use of accessory muscles noted.

Chest: Increased A-P diameter; diminished breath sounds, and diminished heart sounds; Hoover's sign may be present with more severe cases. Bilateral increase in resonance to percussion. Large supraclavicular fossae often present. PMI is difficult to identify or may be felt in the midline area just below the xiphoid process. Patient usually breathes with an increased expiratory time.

Abdomen: Cachexia often present; abdominal paradox present with diaphragm fatigue.

Extremities: Clubbing may or may not be present. Cyanosis uncommon unless an acute pneumonia is present. Pedal edema not usually present unless cor pulmonale is occurring.

Laboratory Data

ABG: Respiratory alkalosis with mild hypoxemia is often present. Respiratory acidosis and severe hypoxemia occur with advanced stages of the disease.

CBC: Not contributory unless an infection is also present. Elevated Hgb may be present.

PFT: Reduced expiratory flow measurements; increased lung volume measurements; reduced DLCO; vital capacity often reduced in proportion with the degree of air trapping.

Chest radiograph: Hyperinflation of the lung fields; large retrosternal airspace seen on the lateral film; low, flat diaphragm; wide rib spacing; increase radiolucency; small narrow heart located midline; diminished vascular markings seen in the bases with alpha$_1$-antitrypsin deficiency.

EKG: Diminished voltage in the limb leads.

TREATMENT

- Assess oxygenation status and correct hypoxemia if present. Usually low-flow oxygen is sufficient.
- Evaluate the patient for evidence of complications (e.g., pneumonia) when indicated by the history of present illness.

- Treat airway obstruction with bronchodilators, especially if a reversible component is present.
- Encourage the patient to enroll in a pulmonary rehabilitation program.
- Encourage the patient to enroll in a smoking cessation program.
- Consult with the attending physician to discuss lung volume reduction surgery if the patient appears to be a candidate.

QUESTIONS FREQUENTLY ASKED BY PATIENT OR CAREGIVER

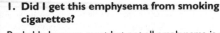

1. Did I get this emphysema from smoking cigarettes?

Probably, because most but not all emphysema is directly or indirectly related to cigarette smoking. A small percentage of patients with emphysema have a genetic cause for their disease. Genetic causes of emphysema may cause it to occur in nonsmokers or at an earlier age (e.g., 30 to 40 years) than in smokers.

2. Is there a cure for emphysema?

No, but most patients feel better with treatment and learn ways to cope with and minimize the symptoms.

3. Why don't the bronchodilators make me feel less short of breath?

Emphysema is a disease caused by destruction of elastic fibers in the lungs. The small airways in the lung tend to collapse during exhalation, which leads to air trapping. The bronchodilators help many patients with emphysema because most also have some component of asthma or bronchospasm that responds to the medication. We cannot be sure who will respond to this medication until it is given. If you do not notice an improvement in your symptoms with the persistent use of your MDI, you should talk to your physician.

4. Can I have a lung transplant?

Lung transplants are not readily available because donors are difficult to find. They are most often done in patients who have severe disease at an early age.

5. Will I get addicted to the oxygen?

You will become no more addicted to oxygen than you are currently addicted to breathing. In other words, no.

6. Why do I get so short of breath when I exert myself?

You get short of breath because you exceed the ability of your lungs to provide an adequate intake of oxygen that is needed during exertion. At rest, your lungs are more able to keep up. Regular exercise may improve your endurance and reduce some of the shortness of breath you experience with exertion.

7. Is it too late to stop smoking?

No. When you stop smoking, the decline in lung function associated with smoking over time is reduced. Most smokers who quit never regain normal lung function, but they do return to the normal rate of lung function decline associated with age.

8. Why is my chest getting so large?

As the lung tissue elasticity is reduced with emphysema, the chest cage protrudes outward.

9. Why do I get so short of breath when I comb my hair?

The muscles of the shoulder are attached to the muscles of breathing. When you lift your arm over your head, the ability of the breathing muscles to function is diminished.

10. Why do I get short of breath when I simply pull on one sock?

Any movement that causes the abdomen to be compressed limits the ability of the diaphragm to function normally. This leads to a diminished ability to breathe normally.

11. Why do I get short of breath after dinner?

A full stomach limits the ability of the diaphragm to move and assist in breathing. Small, more frequent meals are best.

12. Why do I feel less short of breath when I breathe out through pursed lips?

Pursed-lipped breathing causes a slight backpressure in the lung and helps keep small airways open during exhalation. This helps maintain better gas exchange between the lung and the blood for the diffusion of oxygen and carbon dioxide.

13. My doctor tells me I have low oxygen levels in my blood, but I don't feel any better when I use the oxygen. It is very inconvenient; do I really have to use it?

Yes. If your blood oxygen concentration is low, using oxygen will reduce your tendency to develop heart failure and may prolong your life.

14. I get very short of breath easily with exertion, but my oxygen level is too good to qualify for home oxygen therapy. Shouldn't I be on oxygen anyway?

If your oxygen level is adequate during exertion, adding more oxygen will not make your breathing any easier. However, some patients develop low oxygen levels during exertion. Ask your doctor if your oxygen level drops with exertion or if you should be examined for this.

Reference

Wilkins, RL, and Dexter, JR: Respiratory Disease: A Case Study Approach to Patient Care, second edition. FA Davis, Philadelphia, 1998.

Chapter 12

Heart Failure

CHF, also called left ventricular failure, is the failure of the left ventricle to pump blood forward adequately, leading to a buildup of backpressure into the pulmonary circulation. This increase in pulmonary hydrostatic pressure causes fluid to leak out into the interstitial and alveolar spaces of the lung and causes hypoxemia and a reduction in lung compliance.

KEY TERMS

cardiac index–the volume of blood pumped by the left ventricle per minute divided by the body surface area

cardiac output–the volume of blood pumped by the left ventricle per minute

cardiomegaly–enlargement of the heart

diuretic–pharmacologic agent used to assist the kidneys in excreting urine and reducing body fluids

gallop rhythm–an abnormal heart rhythm with added sounds that simulate the gallop of a horse, determined by listening to the heart sounds with a stethoscope

hepatomegaly–enlargement of the liver, usually caused by right HF and engorgement of the hepatic veins

iotropic drugs–medications that assist the heart in pumping blood more forcefully

JVD–abnormal distention of the jugular veins in the neck

orthopnea–the inability to breathe in the supine position, or better breathing in the upright position

paroxysmal nocturnal dyspnea–the sudden onset of dyspnea during the night caused by the gradual buildup of fluid in the lungs

pedal edema–swelling of the ankles caused by a backup of venous blood in the lower extremities

stroke volume–the volume of blood ejected by the left or right ventricle with each contraction

EPIDEMIOLOGY

About 900,000 cases of heart disease are diagnosed each year in the U.S. About 2 to 3 million people in the U.S. have HF.

ETIOLOGY

Most patients with CHF have a history of coronary artery disease in which the arteries are not patent and are unable to provide adequate blood flow to the myocardium. This leads to poor oxygenation of the heart and inadequate pumping of the ventricles. Other causes include chronic hypertension, cardiomyopathy, and valvular defects. Patients can be of any age or ethnicity. Heart disease associated with coronary artery disease is more common in men older than age 45 years and who are obese.

CLINICAL FEATURES

Medical History

Chief Complaints

Chest pain, shortness of breath, nausea, and reduced exercise tolerance.

History of Present Illness

Patient complains of acute SOB and chest pain with a sudden onset often associated with exertion. The pain may radiate to the shoulder, arm, or back. The patient often sleeps with three or more pillows to avoid dyspnea but still may wake up in the middle of the night feeling short of breath.

Past Medical History

Often positive for previous heart problems.

Family History

Often positive for heart disease.

Physical Examination

HEENT: Noncontributory.

Neck: JVD often seen.

Chest: Gallop rhythm with possible murmurs. Adventitious lung sounds are frequently heard. Fine late inspiratory crackles in the dependent regions are most common. Expiratory wheezing may be heard. A ventricular heave may be felt in the left anterior axillary region.

Abdomen: Hepatomegaly.

Extremities: Often show cyanosis and coolness to touch. Pedal edema is common after a day of being in the upright position.

Laboratory Data

ABG: Often show mild to moderate hypoxemia with mild respiratory alkalosis in the early stages of the disease.

ECG: May show elevated ST segments and inverted T waves with tachycardia.

Hemodynamics: Elevated PCWP (>18 mm Hg) is seen with left HF but not when the pulmonary edema is caused by noncardiogenic factors.

Chest radiograph: Shows an enlarged heart with pulmonary edema in the lower lobes. Redistribution of the blood flow to the upper lobes is common in moderate to severe cases. Pleural effusion is seen in some cases when severe HF is present.

TREATMENT

- Reduce pulmonary edema with diuretics.
- Improve oxygenation with oxygen therapy.
- Improve contractility with positive inotropic medications.
- Reduce afterload with vasodilators.

Figure 12–1 outlines the assessment and treatment of pulmonary edema, a major manifestation of HF.

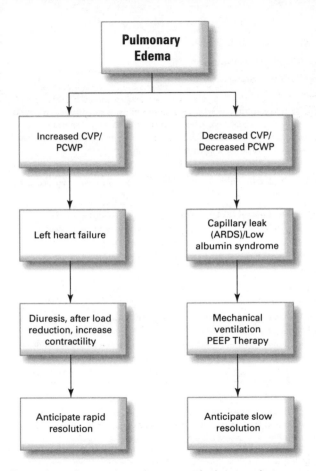

Figure 12–1. *Presentation and treatment of pulmonary edema.*

QUESTIONS FREQUENTLY ASKED BY PATIENT OR CAREGIVER

1. Why do my ankles swell during the day?

A weak heart allows a backpressure to build in the veins that carry blood to the heart. High pressure in these veins results in fluid leaking out into the surrounding tissue. The buildup of high pressure in the blood vessels is most significant in the ankles because this is where gravity has the greatest influence in the upright position.

2. Why am I being given oxygen, how long will I need it, and is it addictive?

You are being given oxygen because your heart needs a good supply of it to work properly. Many patients with HF also have trouble getting adequate oxygen levels into their blood because of fluid that builds up in the lung. Your doctor will determine how long you should be on the oxygen, but it is most common to take it for a few days. Oxygen is not addictive. Be sure you do not smoke or use anything that creates a spark while you are using your oxygen.

3. Will the oxygen explode if I smoke?

No. Oxygen only helps things burn faster; it supports combustion but is not flammable. There have been cases of patients smoking while using oxygen by nasal cannula in which there was a flash type of fire that disfigured the patient's face. In addition, your clothing and bed sheets are prone to the flash type of fire while you are using oxygen.

4. Why do I wake up short of breath at night?

The high backpressure of blood in the veins causes fluid to leak out into surrounding tissues. During the day, this results in ankle swelling because they are the most gravity-dependent regions. During the night, the lungs are very gravity dependent, and gradually fluid leaks out of the pulmonary blood vessels into the lung. This blocks the transfer of oxygen into the blood and causes you to wake up several hours after going to bed with acute shortness of breath.

5. Will I be able to exercise after I go home?

Your doctor will recommend a safe activity level specifically for you at the time of discharge. In general, gentle exercise is good for you.

6. Will my heart be normal again after treatment?

That's a good question for your doctor. In some cases in which HF is mild or caused by a specific cause that can be corrected, your heart should return to normal function. In more severe cases, however, heart function does not return totally to normal.

7. Why do I have to urinate so much?

Fluid collects in the body when the heart is not pumping effectively. Lasix is a diuretic that causes this excess fluid to exit the body through the kidneys and urinary tract. Lasix causes urinary urgency for 3 to 4 hours, so don't take it when you do not have access to a restroom or when you need to be present at a meeting without interruption for a couple of hours. The medication makes you lose potassium, so your doctor may have you take extra potassium to supplement this loss.

8. Why am I so thirsty?

People with HF are often on a diet that restricts that amount of fluid intake. If they also eat salty foods, the combination of limited fluid intake and a high-salt diet leads to extreme sensations of thirst. Talk to your doctor to see if he or she recommends a low-salt diet.

9. My heartbeat is very irregular. What causes this?

CHF causes increased pressures in the right side of the heart, where the pacemaker of the heart is located. This added pressure causes enlargement of the right side of the heart and can lead to stretching of the heart pacemaker and an irregular heart rhythm. You should ask your doctor for more specific information in your case.

10. Is my doctor one of the best in this hospital or should I seek another one?

Your doctor is very qualified and provides excellent care. You are always welcome to get a second opinion from another physician if you so desire.

11. My doctor says I have had an "MI." What is that?

"MI" stands for "myocardial infarction." This indicates that a portion of your heart did not get enough oxygenated blood and the heart tissue experienced damage. If the damaged area is small, you should not have any significant problems. If it is large, your doctor may be able to improve your heart function with medications or a surgical procedure.

12. Why does everyone keep checking my BP?

Your BP is a good indication of how well your heart is working and how much pressure it is generating in the arterial blood system. Pressure that is too low can result in poor perfusion of vital organs, and BP that is too high can put excessive workload on the heart. Several of the medications given to you for your heart also affect your BP. Checking your BP helps us know what therapy is best suited for your case.

13. Why do I keep getting dizzy and feel faint?

Blood flow to your brain is temporarily less than normal. This causes less oxygen to be delivered to your brain, making you feel faint.

References

Haldeman, GA, et al.: Hospitalization of patients with heart failure: National hospital discharge survey, 1985–1995. *Am Heart J* 1999, 137:352–360.

Schocken, DD, et al.: Prevalence and mortality rate of congestive heart failure in the United States. *J Am Coll Cardiol* 1992, 20:301–306.

Wilkins, RL, and Dexter, JR: Respiratory Disease: A Case Study Approach to Patient Care, second edition. FA Davis, Philadelphia, 1998.

Chapter 13

Interstitial Lung Disease

This category of pulmonary disease represents a broad spectrum of conditions that result from a series of events: parenchymal injury, inflammation, disordered tissue repair, fibrotic lung disease, and end-stage lung disease. These conditions may be described according to the presence or absence of granuloma formation or may be referred to as diffuse interstitial infiltrative disorders.

KEY TERMS

hypersensitivity pneumonitis (extrinsic allergic alveolitis)–a pneumonitis caused by the inhalation of organic dusts, certain pharmacologic agents, radiation therapy, and the inhalation of toxic gases (including oxygen), or certain infective agents such as *Thermoactinomyces vulgaris*

idiopathic pulmonary fibrosis–a progressive, inflammatory disease with no known cause

pneumoconioses–occupational diseases related to inhalation of inorganic dust particles; these include anthracosis (coal miner's lung), silicosis (caused by the inhalation of silica dust), and asbestosis (characterized by the presence of ferruginous bodies, asbestos fibers 20 to 150 μ in length that are coated with an iron-based protein)

sarcoidosis–a multiorgan system disease that is 20 times more prevalent in blacks than whites, characterized by a noncaseating granuloma formation with mediastinal lymph node involvement

Wegener's granulomatosis–a granuloma-forming disease of the upper and lower respiratory system associated with glomerulonephritis

EPIDEMIOLOGY

The incidence and prevalence of interstitial disease varies and is usually related to a particular exposure. Sarcoidosis, which is more common in temperate zones than tropical, is more prevalent in blacks than whites and is rare in southeast Asians. Idiopathic pulmonary fibrosis is more common in males between the ages of 50 and 70 years. Twenty percent of cancer patients receiving treatment are likely to develop pulmonary fibrosis, which is a major cause of death.

ETIOLOGY

About one third of interstitial lung disease can be attributed to a known cause. The practitioner should obtain a detailed patient history, including a thorough occupational history. The practitioner should also review the list of medications, especially if the patient has a diagnosis of cancer.

CLINICAL FEATURES

Medical History

Chief Complaint

Progressive dyspnea.

History of Present Illness

History of progressive dyspnea on exertion.

Past Medical History

Noncontributory unless concomitant respiratory or cardiac disease is present.

Family History

Noncontributory.

Occupational and Social History

May be significant for occupational exposure to causative agents.

Physical Examination

The physical examination results may be normal early in the disease, but evidence of cor pulmonale and pulmonary hypertension may be found in later stages. Clubbing is more common in patients with asbestosis and idiopathic pulmonary fibrosis. The complete physical may be contributory if the disease is systemic in origin, such as sarcoidosis.

Laboratory Data

ABG: May be normal, but progressive widening of the A-a gradient is found. Hypoxemia during exercise testing is also a common finding.

PFT: In early stages of disease, PFT may be normal. The most common findings are reduced volumes and capacities. The FEV_1/FVC remains normal because the loss of the FEV_1 is proportional to the loss of vital capacity. Reduced DLCO is indicative of parenchymal destruction as the disease progresses. Lung compliance also decreases. It is common for these values to be monitored in those receiving drugs known to cause interstitial lung disease.

Chest radiograph: The radiograph may present in several ways. High-resolution CT scan helps identify the characteristic changes seen in patients with these diseases:

- Early disease: Normal or with an initial abnormality of a ground-glass appearance
- Later disease: Diffuse bilateral ground-glass appearance
- End stage: Honeycombing

Diffuse infiltrates can be categorized into three types:

- Nodular (presence of small nodes)
- Reticular (presence of lines)
- Reticulonodular (combination of nodes and lines)

Some radiographs may demonstrate patterns specific to a disease:

- Asbestosis: Presence of calcified pleural plaques
- Sarcoidosis: Bilateral hilar lymphadenopathy
- Wegener's granuloma: Cavities and nodules in the lower lobes

Lung biopsy: Helpful in definitive diagnosis

TREATMENT

- Reduce inflammation by removing the cause, if it is known. Prednisone and immunosuppressive drugs such as cyclophosphamide and azathioprine may be used.

Supplemental oxygen therapy should be used to relieve hypoxemia. Lung transplantation has been used for end-stage diseases.

QUESTIONS FREQUENTLY ASKED BY PATIENT OR CAREGIVER

1. I never smoked, yet I have pulmonary fibrosis. How could I develop this disease despite never smoking?

Pulmonary fibrosis may be caused by a large number of different causes; for example, infections, drugs, toxic chemicals, and dusts. Cigarette smoking causes emphysema and chronic bronchitis. These diseases are frequently called COPD. Pulmonary fibrosis is a very different type of lung disease, and cigarette smoking is not a major cause of the disease.

2. My breathing is just fine until I try to walk up a hill or climb stairs. Is there anything that I can do to reduce the shortness of breath I get during exertion?

It is common for patients with pulmonary fibrosis to develop shortness of breath when they exert themselves. Sometimes patients with pulmonary fibrosis develop low oxygen levels when they exercise. The shortness of breath from exertion may be improved if the oxygen level is adequate during exercise. A test to measure your blood oxygen level during exercise will tell you if oxygen would help.

3. The inhalers my wife takes for asthma don't help my breathing when I use them. Why not?

Inhalers treat airway obstruction. Airway obstruction is the primary problem in patients with asthma. Pulmonary fibrosis causes the lungs to get stiff, which makes breathing more difficult. The airways of patients with pulmonary fibrosis are usually not obstructed and do not improve with asthma medications.

4. Is there a chance my lungs will get better?

Ask your doctor. Although a few forms of pulmonary fibrosis improve with appropriate treatment, many forms of the disease do not. If you have a type of pulmonary fibrosis that does not improve with treatment, treatment may still be helpful by stopping the disease from further damaging your lungs.

5. Would a lung transplant help?

A lung transplant may be helpful in most forms of advanced pulmonary fibrosis. Lung transplantation is still very uncommon because of a shortage of donor lungs.

6. My doctor gave me prednisone. Will I have to take this the rest of my life?

Prednisone is frequently given for at least 1 year for pulmonary fibrosis. Prednisone may be discontinued if you do not respond to treatment, if you complete a year of treatment and the pulmonary fibrosis goes into remission, or if you and your doctor decide to try a type of treatment other than prednisone.

7. I am taking a drug my pharmacist says is chemotherapy. Is pulmonary fibrosis a form of cancer?

The destruction of the lungs that occurs with pulmonary fibrosis is caused by the immune system's damaging your lungs. Sometimes low doses of chemotherapy (e.g., cyclophosphamide or azothiaprim) inhibit the immune system just enough to stop the immune system from damaging the lungs further. Pulmonary fibrosis is not a form of cancer.

8. I have heard that pulmonary fibrosis causes scarring in the lungs. I have had scars in my lungs for the last 30 years on my chest radiographs. Does that mean I have pulmonary fibrosis?

Sometimes damage to the lungs from an injury or an infection causes a scar to form in the lung. These types of scars are similar to scars in your skin. They represent a healed injury. After they form, they remain unchanged nearly forever. Pulmonary fibrosis causes progressive scarring of the lungs. The scars caused by pulmonary fibrosis get progressively worse. Scars that have been in your lungs for many years almost certainly indicate a previous injury or infection and not pulmonary fibrosis.

9. Why does my doctor insist on repeating my breathing tests so frequently?

With pulmonary fibrosis, there is often a progressive destruction of the lung. Pulmonary function tests give the doctor a reliable way of determining if significant amounts of additional damage have occurred. Repeated measurements of pulmonary function are commonly done in patients with pulmonary fibrosis, either to determine if the disease is progressive or to gauge how effective therapy is.

10. My doctor wants me to have a biopsy of my lung before I start treatment for pulmonary fibrosis. That sounds like major surgery! Is it always necessary to have a lung biopsy for pulmonary fibrosis?

Many patients with pulmonary fibrosis require a lung biopsy to determine exactly which form of pulmonary fibrosis they have. The results of these biopsies help doctors decide which form of treatment to start and what results to expect from the treatment. If you have misgivings or questions about this procedure, please clarify them with your doctor before you agree to have a lung biopsy.

Reference

Wilkins, RL, and Dexter, JR: Respiratory Disease: A Case Study Approach to Patient Care, second edition. FA Davis, Philadelphia, 1998.

Chapter 14

Lung Cancer

Lung cancer can occur as a primary tumor that originates in the lung or as the result of metastasis from cancer in other body tissues.

Lung cancer is the most common cancer-related cause of death and the second most commonly occurring cancer among men and women. It was estimated that there will be 164,100 new cases of lung cancer in the U.S. in 2000 alone. The rate of lung cancer appears to be declining among white and African-American men in the U.S., but it continues to increase among both white and African-American women. An estimated 156,900 Americans were expected to die because of lung cancer in 2000 (American Lung Association).

KEY TERMS

adenocarcinoma–resembles poorly formed gland tissue; may be primary or metastatic; accounts for 30% of all lung cancers

bronchogenic carcinoma–cancer arising in the bronchi

carcinogen–cancer-causing agent

large cell carcinoma–collection of poorly formed large cells with abundant cytoplasm; accounts for 15% of all lung cancers

metastatic cancer–cancer originating in other tissues

primary lung cancer–cancer arising in the lung

small cell carcinoma–cancer that consists of small cells with scant cytoplasm, usually spreads to distant tissue while tumor is small; accounts for 25% of all lung cancers

squamous cell carcinoma–cancer that resembles skin cells and contains keratin; most commonly arises from bronchial lining; accounts for 25% of all lung cancers

staging—method for classifying severity of cancer based on nature of the primary tumor, the lymph node involvement, and metastasis (TNM system)

EPIDEMIOLOGY

Most common fatal cancer in men and women, accounting for 32% of cancer deaths in men and 25% in women.

ETIOLOGY

Strong association with cigarette smoking and secondary cigarette smoke exposure. Other carcinogens include asbestos, chromium, radon, and nickel.

CLINICAL FEATURES

Medical History

Chief Complaints

Cough, hemoptysis, weight loss, dyspnea.

History of Present Illness

Patient may be asymptomatic or complain of change in nature of cough or sputum production. Unresolving or recurrent pneumonia may be present.

Past Medical History

Noncontributory.

Family History

Familial history predisposes patient to increased susceptibility.

Occupational and Social History

History of cigarette smoking or occupational exposure to a known carcinogen.

Physical Examination

May be normal in patients with small tumors.

Vital Signs: Normal or tachypnea.

Sensorium: Normal.

HEENT: Normal.

Neck: Normal or lymphadenopathy.

Chest:

Inspection: Normal.

Palpation: Normal.

Percussion: Normal or dull over area of a large tumor or atelectatic area or pneumonia or effusion.

Auscultation: Normal or monophonic wheezing, rhonchi.

Abdomen: Normal.

Extremities: Normal or clubbing.

Laboratory Data

ABG: Normal or respiratory alkalosis with mild hypoxemia.

PFT: Normal or decreased volumes and flow rates depending on size and location of the tumor. Preoperative evaluation important in determining risk and pulmonary reserve.

Chest radiograph: Normal or presence of nodule, pneumonia, atelectasis, or pleural effusion.

Other data:

Sputum: Cytology may be helpful.

Bronchoscopy: Washings, brushings, and forceps biopsy.

TREATMENT

Depends on histology of the tumor. Surgical resection (i.e., lobectomy or pneumonectomy) provides the only chance for cure. Radiation can be palliative for patients with hemoptysis or bone metastasis. Chemotherapy is indicated for those with small cell carcinoma. Oxygen therapy and bronchodilators may help alleviate associated symptoms.

Figure 14–1 outlines the types of lung mass and their treatment.

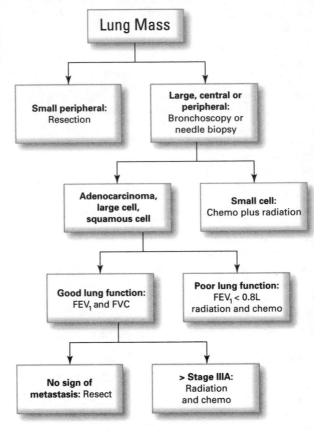

Figure 14–1. *Types and treatment of lung masses.*

QUESTIONS FREQUENTLY ASKED BY PATIENT OR CAREGIVER

1. If I quit smoking, can I still get lung cancer?

Yes. The risk goes down each year you don't smoke but will never reach the same risk level as that of a nonsmoker.

2. Is there a cure for lung cancer?

Small lung cancers are curable if they have clear borders and have not spread to other areas of the body. Cancers that have spread can be treated but are more difficult to cure. You should ask your doctor for more details about your specific case.

3. How many different types of lung cancer exist?

Four common types of lung cancer exist: small cell, large cell, squamous cell, and adenocarcinoma. The type of cancer present often dictates which therapy will be used to treat the lung cancer. You should talk to your physician about your specific case.

4. How will my doctor know if surgery is possible?

A tumor surrounded by healthy lung tissue that has not spread to other sites can usually be removed by surgery. Pulmonary function tests should be done to determine your current pulmonary status and how well you might respond to removal of a portion of your lungs.

5. What is a hospice?

A hospice is a team of healthcare professionals who work to provide comfort and dignity for people with a terminal illness. Hospice is usually reserved for patients in their last 6 months of life. A periodic evaluation by your attending physician is useful to determine the best time to start such a program for you.

6. Will I have pain with the lung cancer?

Each case is different, and lung cancer may or may not cause you pain. The location of the cancerous tumor is a key issue because abnormal growths near the outer edge of the lung often involve the pleura, which is associated with more painful breathing. Fortunately, very good pain medications exist, so pain can almost always be controlled.

7. How long will I live?

That is a very difficult question to answer. Even the most experienced doctors have a difficult time accurately predicting life expectancy. Variables such as the aggressiveness of the cancer and preexisting health condition are two major factors that predict life expectancy. All the published literature is based on large groups of people, so a study predicting an average 2-year life expectancy is made up of half the people who did not live 2 years and half who lived longer.

8. I have noticed a new pain in my back (or leg). Should I ask my doctor about it?

You definitely need to notify your doctor about this new pain. Such information may influence the treatment program your doctor is planning.

9. I suddenly got extremely hoarse after being diagnosed with a lung cancer. Is there a possible connection?

There is a long nerve that loops from the neck around the aorta in the left side of your chest and controls your left vocal cord. If the lung tumor is near your heart or aorta, it could pinch off the nerve and cause a change in the quality of your voice tones. Ask your doctor if this could be the cause.

10. I have smoked cigarettes for the past 34 years and now I have been told I may have lung cancer. Is the lung cancer a result of my smoking habit?

It is impossible to say that cigarettes caused your lung cancer, but smokers do have a higher risk for lung cancer than do nonsmokers. Some studies have shown longer survival time for cancer patients who stopped smoking, so it is wise to participate in a smoking cessation program as soon as possible.

11. What is chemotherapy?

Chemotherapy is the administration of numerous chemical agents that fight cancer cells. Most of the chemotherapy is given by a combination of oral and IV routes. It is not painful, but side effects (e.g., nausea and vomiting) are common.

12. Why did the respiratory therapist ask for a sputum specimen?

The sputum specimen will be sent to the laboratory for analysis. This analysis can be helpful in determining what type of cancer you have and if any infection is occurring.

13. What is radiation therapy?

It is a therapy that applies high doses of radiation to the cancer or tumor to try to kill the cancer cells.

References

American Lung Association. *http://beta.lungusa.org/diseases/lungcanc.html*
Braun, SR, et al: Concise Textbook of Pulmonary Medicine. Elsevier, New York, 1989.
Wilkins, RL, and Dexter, JR: Respiratory Disease: A Case Study Approach to Patient Care, second edition. FA Davis, Philadelphia, 1998.

Chapter 15

Near-Drowning

Near-drowning is a term applied to the status of people who are successfully resuscitated after submersion in a liquid for a significant period of time. The outcome is highly variable and related to the time of submersion, water temperature, and quality of emergency life support applied after the patient is resuscitated.

KEY TERMS

anaerobic metabolism–metabolism without oxygen

aspiration–inhalation of foreign material into the lungs

drowning–death by suffocation resulting from submersion in water or any liquid

dry drowning–suffocation by drowning without aspiration

hypoxia–a significant decrease in the presence of oxygen at the tissue level

lactic acid–the substance produced by anaerobic metabolism

persistent vegetative state–the state that occurs after a person has been resuscitated after submersion but has permanent brain damage

wet drowning–a drowning in which the victim aspirates water into the lungs

EPIDEMIOLOGY

A total of 150,000 deaths occur worldwide each year because of drowning, with 6000 to 8000 occurring in the U.S.

Approximately 80,000 near-drowning events occur each year in the U.S. The highest incidence of drowning occurs in children under the age of 5 years and in teenage boys.

ETIOLOGY

Not applicable.

CLINICAL FEATURES

Medical History

The clinical features of near-drowning victims vary widely depending on the length of submersion and subsequent degree of brain damage.

Chief Complaints

Not applicable.

History of Present Illness

Recent history of catastrophic event.

Family History

Not applicable.

Occupational and Social History

Not applicable.

Physical Examination

In most cases, the patient is unconscious with unstable vital signs. The pulse rate may be absent, fast, or slow. The respiratory rate is usually controlled by the resuscitation team with a bag valve mask or endotracheal tube. BP is important to monitor and is typically low. Body temperature should be measured and is a reflection of the water temperature and duration of submersion.

HEENT: Pupils may be dilated and minimally responsive or nonresponsive to light. The neck should be inspected for evidence of trauma caused by diving into shallow water.

Chest: Auscultation may reveal coarse crackles if the patient has aspirated. Heart sound may be absent if resuscitation is occurring. It is important to inspect for evidence of respiratory effort periodically because it indicates improvement.

Abdomen: May be distended from air or water.

Extremities: Often cool to the touch with poor capillary refill.

Chest radiograph: Should be inspected for evidence of gastric aspiration and ARDS.

TREATMENT

The initial treatment of all near-drowning victims is to activate the EMS system and begin CPR. After the patient is stable and transferred to a medical center, treatment depends on the response of the patient to CPR. Most victims are intubated and placed on controlled mechanical ventilation. Treatment should be aimed at providing good oxygenation, ventilation, BP level, and electrolyte balance. The intracranial pressure should be kept normal. This may require hyperventilation and close monitoring of hemodynamics.

QUESTIONS FREQUENTLY ASKED BY PATIENT OR CAREGIVER

1. Will my child be normal?

I cannot answer that question. You will have to ask the doctor.

2. Why is my child on the ventilator?

Your child's submersion accident created abnormalities in the function of his or her lungs. These changes made oxygenation of his or her blood less efficient. The ventilator helps the lungs better oxygenate the blood, making it easier for your child to breathe.

3. Does my child have pneumonia?

Not at this time. Most of the lung injury is a result of aspirated water. However, bacterial infection of his or her lungs may occur. We will be watching for signs of pneumonia. If these signs are found, your doctor will immediately implement the appropriate treatment.

4. Will my child's lungs get better?

Most likely they will, but it may take days. However, pulmonary deterioration may occur during your child's treatment. You should ask your doctor to explain your child's current lung function as well as keep you updated on the lungs' recovery.

5. Will the ventilator damage my child's lungs?

The ventilator supports the lungs until they heal. Occasionally, the pressure required to push the gas into the lung does cause some injury. Usually this lung injury resolves with time and is not a major concern.

6. Will my child become dependent on the ventilator?

In almost all cases, children are able to be weaned (come off) from the ventilator.

7. How long will my child be on the ventilator?

I cannot answer that with confidence; it depends on the rate of recovery and any complications that occur. You may want to ask your doctor to see if he or she has a better answer.

8. Why does my child need oxygen?

Aspiration of fluid into the airway triggers a series of events. The primary effect is to disrupt the lungs' ability to effectively take in oxygen. We can overcome this problem by giving your child additional oxygen to breathe.

9. What is that noise my child made when you took out the endotracheal tube?

That noise is called stridor. It results from swelling in the trachea caused by the endotracheal tube. It usually goes away within 24 hours or less. We will be keeping an eye on this to make sure it does not become a problem.

10. Can I hold my child while he or she is on the ventilator?

At times, physicians allow that to occur. Before we allow it, however, we should check with your child's doctor.

11. Why is my child so stiff?

This occurs in some children after these accidents. The stiffness sometimes interferes with treatment, such as the breathing machine, and the physician will provide medication to decrease the stiffness. You should also ask your doctor about this.

12. Is my child in pain?

No, not to our knowledge. The physicians and nurses are careful to take care of childhood pain. If you have more questions about pain, I recommend asking your doctor.

References

Bolle, R: Drowning: A preventable cause of death. Contemp Pediatr 1999, 16:94–115.

DeNicola, LK, et al.: Submersion injuries in children and adults. Crit Care Clin 1997, 13:477–502.

Quan, L. Near-drowning. Pediatr Rev 1999, 20:255–259.

Wilkins, RL, and Dexter, JR: Respiratory Disease: A Case Study Approach to Patient Care, second edition. FA Davis, Philadelphia, 1998.

Chapter 16

Neuromuscular Disease

This grouping of diseases can be categorized into four distinct classes, as shown in Table 16–1.

KEY TERMS

diplopia–double vision

fasciculations–involuntary fine tremor of muscle fibers

paresthesia–a sensation of numbness or tingling in central or peripheral nerve endings

ptosis–drooping of the eyelids

EPIDEMIOLOGY

Epidemiologic factors for the different diseases include age, gender, and history of viral infection.

ETIOLOGY

The etiology of neuromuscular disease varies. The cause of ALS has yet to be discovered, but it is known that Guillain-Barré syndrome is often preceded by a viral illness. Trauma is the most common cause of spinal cord disorders.

CLINICAL FEATURES

Clinical features are dependent on the nature of the disorder.

Medical History
Chief Complaint

Table 16–1 *Classification of Neuromuscular Disorders*

Location of Defect	Disorder
CNS	Ondine's curse Central sleep apnea Primary alveolar hypoventilation Sedative hypnotic overdose
Neuronal pathway	Spinal cord injury MS ALS Guillain-Barré syndrome
Neuromuscular junction	Myasthenia gravis Botulism poisoning Organophosphate poisoning
Muscular function	MD Myotonic dystrophy

From Wilkins, RL, and Dexter, JR: Respiratory Disease: A Case Study Approach to Patient Care, second edition. FA Davis, Philadelphia, 1998, p. 307; with permission

The client may complain of muscle weakness, shortness of breath on exertion or during rest, difficulty swallowing, or, in the case of those with ALS, fasciculations.

History of Present Illness

There may or may not have been a previous viral-type illness that would suggest Guillain-Barré syndrome. If the client has sustained a spinal cord injury, the nature, level, and completeness of the injury is significant.

Past Medical History

Noncontributory unless the disease is congenital or the patient has a history of pulmonary disease that may complicate respiratory care.

Family History

Noncontributory.

Occupational and Social History

Noncontributory except for smoking history.

Physical Examination

Vital Signs: Normal except for tachypnea.

Sensorium: Normal.

HEENT: Look for ptosis or evidence of diplopia. Difficulty speaking or swallowing may be noted.

Neck: Normal.

Chest:

Inspection: Normal.

Palpation: Normal.

Percussion: Normal.

Auscultation: Decreased breath sounds bilaterally; râles or rhonchi may be present.

Abdomen: Normal.

Extremities: Normal or presence of fasciculations, muscle weakness, or wasting. Presence of paresthesias may be found in patients with Guillain-Barré syndrome. Observe the client for dysarthria.

Laboratory Data

ABG: Mild to moderate hypoxemia. Respiratory acidosis is the primary acid-base disturbance in patients with advanced disease.

PFT: Decreased volumes and capacities. Vital capacity of less than 10 to 15 mL/kg and maximum inspiratory pressures less than -20 cm H_2O may indicate the need for ventilatory support. Establishment of a baseline and continued trend monitoring is indicated in determining the progression of the disease.

Chest radiograph: Hypoinflation.

Other data:

Tensilon test: Positive result indicates myasthenia gravis.

Video swallowing study: Determines the client's risk of aspiration.

Electromyelogram: Helpful in determining decreased transmission at the neuromuscular junction.

Lumbar puncture: Increased protein in those with Guillain-Barré syndrome.

TREATMENT

For respiratory care practitioners, the care of a patient with neuromuscular disease involves pulmonary toileting and ventilatory support. Modalities such as nebulized bronchodilators and mucolytics, IPPV or other devices, postural drainage, "quad" coughing, hyperinflation by manual insufflation, or use of the insufflator or exsufflator are all appropriate for removing or preventing retained secretions.

The choice of using an artificial airway and ventilatory support is based on the client's wishes. The inability to cough out secretions and a high risk of aspiration are the determining factors for the need for an artificial airway. The inability to maintain acid-base balance indicates the need for ventilatory support. Ventilatory support can be achieved noninvasively or invasively.

QUESTIONS FREQUENTLY ASKED BY PATIENT OR CAREGIVER

1. I thought that breathing muscles were different than other muscles and were not affected by a muscle disease.

No. Breathing muscles are affected by muscle diseases just like any other muscle.

2. I have paraplegia from an accident. Since the accident, I can't cough as effectively as I used to. Is there anything that can be done to help this?

Coughing is the result of a series of actions. You take a deep breath, close your vocal cords, and then build up pressure in your lungs just before you open your vocal cords and complete the cough. Many patients with paraplegia cannot build pressure in their lungs because the nerves that supply the muscles of their abdomen do not work. As a result, the cough seems weak and ineffective. Having someone press on the abdomen during a cough helps increase the pressure in your lungs and makes the cough more effective.

3. I have quadraplegia at the C3–4 level. For many months now, I have been able to breathe on my own during the day and use a ventilator only at night. Because I recently developed pneumonia, I must use the ventilator nearly all the time. Will I ever be able to breathe on my own again?

Many patients with quadriplegia may breathe on their own for periods of time. In order to breathe, they rely on the muscles of the neck and shoulder that still function. Breathing using the muscles of the neck and shoulders is effective for minutes to hours. When an infection such as pneumonia affects the lungs, the lungs become stiffer. This change is usually temporary. As the lungs recover, the amount of time you can breathe on your own will usually increase.

4. My doctor says my ALS has worsened to the point where I will need a ventilator or I will die. He told me there were two ways of using a ventilator, either through a mask or a tube in my throat. Could you explain this to me.

When mechanical ventilation is required for patients with ALS, it can be delivered two ways, either by a mask covering your nose or face or by surgically inserting a tube through the skin in your neck into the windpipe. Using a mask has the advantage that it can easily be removed if the ventilator is not required, and it does not require surgery to place. Unfortunately, mask ventilation becomes less effective as the muscles become weaker. If mask ventilation becomes less effective, if you wish, a tube can be placed into your windpipe to provide a more secure means of providing ventilation.

5. You keep pushing this machine (spirometer) into my face and asking me to blow in it. I have something wrong with my muscles and I am weak and tired. Can't you just go away!?

Yes, I suppose I could go away, but that wouldn't help you or your doctor decide if your muscles are strong enough for you to breathe on your own. With many forms of muscle weakness, the muscles may become so weak that you can't breathe effectively. Repeatedly measuring your lung function allows your doctor to monitor the strength of your respiratory muscles. As long as your breathing muscles are strong, you can safely breathe on your own. If your muscles weaken, you may need help with your breathing from a ventilator. By measuring your breathing strength repeatedly, we can identify respiratory muscle weakness before it has serious consequences.

6. My doctor said that to help my breathing, I need to lose weight. Is there really any relationship between my weight and my breathing?

Yes, weight does affect breathing in some overweight patients. If being overweight is causing breathing problems, losing weight usually helps correct the problem.

7. Ever since my father's stroke, he has had one episode of pneumonia after another. Could there be a relationship between the stroke and these episodes of pneumonia?

Some patients who develop strokes don't control their swallowing well. Sometimes when they swallow, some of the material they are trying to swallow goes into the lungs. We call this "aspiration." Each time someone aspirates, they may get pneumonia. One of the causes of repeated pneumonia is recurrent aspiration. An easy test to perform is a video swallowing evaluation to see if he is aspirating.

8. If my father is aspirating, what can be done about it?

Check with your doctor. There is a wide range of options, from modifying the diet to placing a feeding tube into his stomach. The best approach for your father's aspiration is based on the severity and the circumstances surrounding the aspiration.

9. My 3-year-old son was just diagnosed with muscular dystrophy. His breathing seems fine, but I understand he will need a ventilator in the future. How will I know when he needs to start using a ventilator?

Your doctor will monitor the strength of your son's respiratory muscles and the level of carbon dioxide and oxygen in his blood. There are usually several months' warning that the time to begin mechanical ventilation is approaching. Your doctor will see changes in the parameters he is monitoring and let you know if your son's breathing is being compromised.

10. My ventilator is set with an inspiratory pressure of 16 cm of water and an expiratory pressure of 12 cm of water. I don't feel I'm getting enough air. How can I feel better?

Most changes in the ventilator are based on a blood gas. If you have not had a blood gas determination recently, It should be checked. If you aren't getting enough air with each breath, increasing the inspiratory pressure should give you more air with each breath.

References

Braun SR, et al. Concise Textbook of Pulmonary Medicine. Elsevier, New York, 1989.

Wilkins, RL, and Dexter, JR: Respiratory Disease: A Case Study Approach to Patient Care, second edition. FA Davis, Philadelphia, 1998.

Chapter 17

Persistent Pulmonary Hypertension of the Newborn

PPHN is caused by any pulmonary or cardiac disease that results in increased pulmonary vascular resistance by pulmonary vasoconstriction (e.g., acute diseases such as infection, hypoglycemia, polycythemia, short-term placental insufficiency), increased pulmonary vascular musculature (e.g., chronic intrauterine hypoxia), or decreased cross-sectional area of pulmonary vasculature (e.g., pulmonary hypoplasia, congenital diaphragmatic hernia).

KEY TERMS

ECMO–a modality of oxygenating the blood by removing the venous blood with a catheter and passed by a membrane oxygenator; the oxygenated blood is then warmed and returned into the infant's arterial system

maladaptation–the lack of appropriate physiologic changes to extrauterine life

nitric oxide (NO)–a pharmacologic gas that achieves pulmonary vasodilatation when administered in low doses

PFC–failure of the fetal circulation to make the transition to neonatal circulation; manifested by right-to-left shunting of blood across a patent foramen ovale or a PDA

EPIDEMIOLOGY

Usually seen in post-term infants; the incidence varies but is related to risk factors. PPHN has a high mortality rate.

ETIOLOGY

Maladaptation to extrauterine life resulting in acidemia and chronic hypoxemia, meconium aspiration, diaphragmatic hernia, atelectasis, and pneumonia.

CLINICAL FEATURES

Post-term infant, possibly with no respiratory distress at birth; PFC may be present.

Medical History

Chief Complaint

Hypoxemia.

History of Present Illness

Normal delivery with no history of respiratory distress, but one or more of the associated risk factors.

Past Medical History

Not applicable.

Family History

Presence of maternal risk factors.

Occupational and Social History

Presence of maternal risk factors.

Physical Examination

Cyanosis.

Vital signs: Tachycardia and tachypnea with periods of apnea.

Sensorium: Neurologic impairment: seizures, poor muscle tone, poor posture and reflexes.

HEENT: Possible nasal flaring.

Neck: Normal.

Chest:

Inspection: Normal or subcostal or intercostal retractions.

Percussion: Prominent right ventricle.

Auscultation: Normal breath sounds; murmur may be present; loud S2, P2, with narrow S2 split.

Abdomen: Normal.

Extremities: Cyanosis may be present.

Laboratory Data

ABG: Severe hypoxemia that is unresponsive to oxygen therapy. Pre- and postductal pulse oximetry is useful for identifying significant right-to-left shunts across the ductus arteriosus. Hyperoxia test is used to determine oxygen responsiveness.

PFT: Not performed.

Chest radiography: Decreased pulmonary vascular markings. May have right ventricular hypertrophy.

Other data: ECG with Doppler for presence of right-to-left shunt across PDA or persistent patent foramen ovale.

TREATMENT

Decrease vascular resistance: Induced alkalosis (hyperventilation or bicarbonate infusion), oxygen, tolazoline, nitric oxide; ECMO is used when conventional methods fail.

QUESTIONS FREQUENTLY ASKED BY PATIENT OR CAREGIVER

1. Is this disease fatal?

This disease has a high mortality rate but is not usually fatal.

2. Will my child have long-term lung damage?

Most infants who survive this disease will have completely normal lungs. However, because of the severity of this disease and the frequently heroic interventions necessary to save these infants' lives, some infants may develop chronic lung disease or bronchopulmonary dysplasia.

3. Are there any other long-term complications?

Most infants with this disease will not have other long-term complications. However, infants with underlying anatomic causes for PPHN (e.g., congenital diaphragmatic hernia or congenital heart disease) may have other problems related to these other diseases that show up in other organ systems. You should talk with your baby's doctor for specifics about your baby.

4. Will my child have any learning disabilities?

Most children who recover from PPHN will be completely normal and will not have any learning disabilities. However, infants who have very severe disease may suffer injury to their CNS that could lead to learning disabilities.

5. Will my child be able to live a normal life?

Most children who survive PPHN will lead completely normal lives. Some children who have other underlying diseases as the cause for PPHN (e.g., congenital diaphragmatic hernia or congenital heart disease) may have problems related to their underlying disease. If you have specific questions about your baby's condition, be sure to talk to his or her doctor.

6. If I have any more children, will they get this as well?

No, usually PPHN is unique to an individual infant. It is not inherited or passed on in families.

7. Is there anything I could have done during my pregnancy to have prevented this?

No. None of the causes for this disease are preventable by altering pregnancy care.

8. Is it hereditary?

No. It is not inherited or passed on in families.

9. Will the child require care at home?

Probably not. Most infants who survive PPHN are normal. Occasionally, some infants who have other underlying diseases or have had a very severe form of the PPHN do require various types of home care. If you have questions about your baby, ask his or her doctor.

10. Is my child at greater risk for developing SIDS?

No. Infants who survive PPHN are not at higher risk for SIDS.

Reference

Wilkins RL, Dexter JR: Respiratory Disease: A Case Study Approach to Patient Care, second edition. FA Davis, Philadelphia, 1998.

Chapter 18

Pneumonia

Pneumonia is an infection of the lung parenchyma. It may be caused by bacterial, viral, or fungal organisms (see Chapter 19) and may cause severe interference with gas exchange. The degree of lung involved and the underlying condition of the patient often determine the ultimate outcome.

KEY TERMS

bacterial pneumonia–infection of the lung caused by bacteria; can be categorized as community acquired or nosocomial

pneumonitis–inflammation of the lung caused by infection or inhalation of toxic gases

viral pneumonia–pneumonia caused by a viral agent

EPIDEMIOLOGY

Although pneumonia can occur at any age and in all groups, predisposing factors may aid in determining the cause and treatment. These factors are age, impaired gag reflex or lack of cough, immunosuppressive disease, and chronic lung disease. Invasive procedures such as endotracheal intubation, mechanical ventilation, and poor infection control practices are the causes of nosocomial pneumonia.

ETIOLOGY

Pneumonia can be caused by a wide variety of organisms. Common causes of bacterial pneumonia are:

- *Streptococcus pneumoniae.*
- *Hemophilus influenzae.*
- *Mycoplasma pneumonia.*
- *Klebsiella pneumoniae, Enterobacter* spp., and *Legionella pneumophila* are causes associated with aspiration.

- *Pneumocystis carinii* is found predominantly in patients with AIDS.
- *Staphylococcus aureus* and *Pseudomonas aeruginosa* are implicated in nosocomial infections.
- "Atypical" pneumonias are not bacterial in origin.
- Viruses.
- Fungi: Histoplasmosis, coccidioidomycosis, aspergillus, and blastomycosis (see Chapter 19).

CLINICAL FEATURES

Medical History

Chief Complaint

Most common complaints are fever, chills, cough, increased sputum production, dyspnea, and chest pain.

History of Present Illness

Patients complain of the onset or worsening of symptoms for a week or more. History of organ transplant or invasive procedures may indicate the presence of a nosocomial infection. Fungal infections are diagnosed based on exposure history and isolation of the organism (see Chapter 19).

Past Medical History

History of predisposing factors may help in determining origin and treatment.

Family History

Noncontributory.

Occupational and Social History

Noncontributory except for cigarette smoking.

Physical Examination

Assess overall appearance. Accessory muscle use may be present.

Vital signs: Presence of fever, tachycardia, and tachypnea. BP is essentially normal.

Sensorium: Essentially alert to person, place, and time.

HEENT: Normal except for the possible presence of cyanosis of the oral mucosa. Mucous membranes may be dehydrated.

Neck: Normal with the possible presence of cervical and supraclavicular lymphadenopathy.

Chest:

Inspection: Generally normal in appearance with decreased excursion on the affected side.

Palpation: Increased tactile fremitus over the affected area.

Percussion: Diminished or dull note over the affected area.

Auscultation: Diminished in the affected area, pleural friction rub may be present.

Abdomen: Normal.

Extremities: Cyanosis or poor skin turgor caused by dehydration may be present. No clubbing or absence of pulses noted.

Laboratory Data

ABG: Normal acid-base balance or respiratory alkalosis, with mild to moderate hypoxemia.

PFT: Not performed.

Chest radiograph: Lobar or patchy, segmental infiltrates (bronchopneumonia).

Other data:

CBC: Leukocytosis. May be normal in mycoplasma or nonbacterial pneumonia.

Sputum Gram stain: Aids in determining choice of antibiotic.

Sputum C&S: May be beneficial only if an adequate sputum sample is obtained.

TREATMENT

Treatment may be on an outpatient or inpatient basis (see Figure 18–1).

- Antibiotics: Empirical treatment, or antibiotic based on laboratory findings, is the first-line treatment. Penicillin is used

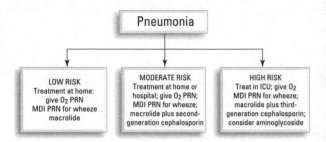

Figure 18–1.   *Treatment of pneumonia.*

for gram-positive organisms, and ampicillin or second-generation cephalosporins are used for gram-negative organisms.

- Oxygen therapy to alleviate hypoxemia. Antipyretics for fever. Adequacy of systemic hydration should also be assessed.
- Bronchodilators may be indicated.

Table 18–1 summarizes the presentation and treatment of pneumonia.

QUESTIONS FREQUENTLY ASKED BY PATIENT OR CAREGIVER

1. Are my lungs permanently damaged?

Not likely, because pneumonia rarely causes permanent damage to the lungs.

2. Am I likely to get pneumonia again?

Not unless there is an underlying problem or immune system deficiency. Consult your physician.

3. Should I get the pneumonia vaccination?

Yes, especially if you are over the age of 55 years or have a history of lung disease.

Table 18-1 Summary of Presentation and Treatment of Pneumonia

Cause	History	Physical Examination	Chest Radiography	Laboratory Findings	Medication
Pneumococcus	Abrupt onset: Chills, fever, cough	Rales, rhonchi, consolidation	Lobar, bronchopneumonia	Gram positive	Penicillin erythromycin
Anaerobes	Aspiration syndromes	Rales, rhonchi, consolidation	Infiltrates in dependent lobes	Mixed flora	Penicillin
Mycoplasma	Frequently mild; more common in young adults	Rales	Patchy consolidation, bronchopneumonia	Serology levels	Erythromycin
Legionella	Gradual onset, headache, chills, fever, cough	Rales, rhonchi	Alveolar infiltrates	Serology levels	Erythromycin
H. influenzae	Acute onset: Chills, fever, cough	Rales, rhonchi	Lobar, bronchopneumonia	Gram negative	Ampicillin, cephalosporins

continued

Pneumonia

Table 18–1 Summary of Presentation and Treatment of Pneumonia (Continued)

Cause	History	Physical Examination	Chest Radiography	Laboratory Findings	Medication
S. aureus	Acute onset: Toxic, fever, cough	Rales	Effusions, multiple areas of consolidation	Gram positive	Vancomycin
Gram negative	Acute onset: Toxic, fever, cough	Rales, rhonchi, consolidation	Lobar, cavitation	Gram negative	Cephalosporin
Viral	Fever, dyspnea, dry cough, more common in winter	Rales, consolidation	Diffuse infiltrates, bilateral	—	—
Fungal	Exposure	Rales, rhonchi, consolidation	Lobar	Isolation of organism	Amphotericin B

Adapted from Braun, SR, et al. Concise Textbook of Pulmonary Medicine. Elsevier, New York, 1989, pp. 192–193.

4. How can I protect myself from getting pneumonia again?

Proper rest, exercise, and diet are essential in maintaining good health. Smoking cigarettes increases the likelihood of pneumonia. You should stop smoking if you smoke.

5. What is walking pneumonia?

Pneumonia that is not severe enough to require bedrest is often called "walking pneumonia."

6. How long do I take the antibiotics?

You should follow the directions on the label very carefully. Many patients stop taking the antibiotics when they feel better and relapse soon thereafter. Most antibiotics are given for about 10 days.

7. How soon should my chest radiograph clear up?

It is difficult to say exactly, but young, previously healthy people usually have a clear radiograph 2 to 3 weeks after onset. Patients with COPD who are elderly may not have a clear radiograph for several months.

8. Is my pneumonia contagious?

It may be mildly contagious. Tell your visitors to wash their hands after any contact with you. Other than that, there is no need for precautions unless it is otherwise stated by your physician. Visitors with suppressed immune systems should wear a mask.

9. My pneumonia has cleared up, but I still cough and wheeze. Why?

Lung infection is a strong inflammatory stimulus and causes persistent inflammation of the airways in some patients. Many patients cough and wheeze for months after the acute infection has cleared. Contact your physician if you think your symptoms are increasing.

10. Why does it hurt when I cough or take a deep breath?

Pneumonia at the edge of the lung irritates the sensitive lining of the lung and may cause a sharp pain with any maneuver that causes the lung lining to move significantly.

Reference

Wilkins, RL, Dexter, JR: Respiratory Disease: A Case Study Approach to Patient Care, second edition. FA Davis, Philadelphia, 1998.

Chapter 19

Pneumonia, Fungal

Fungal pneumonia is inflammation of the lung parenchyma caused by infection with a fungus. It often occurs in patients with compromised immune systems.

 KEY TERMS

autoimmune disease–disease such as arthritis, lupus erythematosus, or scleroderma in which the immune system attacks the host

fungus–an eukaryotic organism that lacks chlorophyll and reproduces by budding or spore formation; there are about 100 fungi common in humans, and 10 can cause disease

neutropenia–abnormal decrease in the number of neutrophils

opportunistic infection–infection caused by organisms that usually does not affect individuals with normal immune systems

EPIDEMIOLOGY

Fungal pneumonias are not common in ordinary individuals, and predisposing factors aid in determining the cause and treatment. The main factors are a history of immunosuppression such as AIDS, use of immunosuppressive drugs for treating arthritis and lupus, neutropenia after chemotherapy, and after organ transplantation. It is very important that clinicians obtain a thorough medical history. In clients with AIDS or other immunosuppression, multiple infective agents, thus complicating the diagnosis and treatment, can cause the pneumonia.

ETIOLOGY

- Aspergillus: Usually associated with exposure to decaying plant matter such as leaves or compost.
- Histoplasmosis: A fungus common in the Mississippi River Valley. Airborne spores from infected bird droppings spread it.
- Coccidioidomycosis: Also spread by airborne spores, this fungal infection is endemic in warm dry areas such as the American Southwest and is usually associated with AIDS. Also known as desert fever, San Joaquin fever, and valley fever.
- *Candida* spp.: A common fungus found in the mucous membranes. It can cause minor infections in healthy individuals and major infection in immunocompromised patients.
- *Cryptococcus neoformans:* A commonly found fungus that can normally exist in the soil and on hands of individuals who are well. Infection is associated with individuals with immuno-suppression.
- Blastomycosis: Usually found in the American Southeast, this fungus is more common in young men living in that geographic area. Also called Gilchrist's disease.

CLINICAL FEATURES

Medical History

Chief Complaint

Most common complaints are fever, chills, cough, increased sputum production, dyspnea, and chest pain. Some patients may also complain of night sweats, loss of appetite, and weight loss.

History of Present Illness

Patients complain of the onset or worsening of symptoms for a week or more. Fungal infections can be suspected if the other causative agents of pneumonia have been ruled out or there is a history of organ transplant or chemotherapy. Exposure history, including travel to areas known to be endemic for fungal infection, and isolation of the organism are also important in making the diagnosis of fungal pneumonia.

Past Medical History

History of HIV, autoimmune disease, and organ transplantation longer than 1 month before onset; chemotherapy; and travel to suspected areas may be helpful in determining the cause and treatment.

Family History

Noncontributory.

Occupational and Social History

Noncontributory except for cigarette smoking or for exposure to decaying vegetation. Recent travel to endemic areas.

Physical Examination

Assess overall appearance. Client may appear to be chronically ill with noticeable weight loss.

Vital signs: Presence of fever that may be low grade and tachypnea. BP and heart rate are essentially normal.

Sensorium: Essentially alert to person, place, and time.

HEENT: Oral mucosa may be normal or with candidiasis, whitish plaque may be seen on the tongue and palate.

Neck: Cervical and supraclavicular lymphadenopathy may be present.

Chest:

Inspection: Generally normal in appearance.

Palpation: Normal.

Percussion: Normal.

Auscultation: Diminished in the affected area, pleural friction rub may be present.

Abdomen: Normal.

Extremities: Normal.

Laboratory Data.

ABG: Normal acid-base balance or respiratory alkalosis, with mild to moderate hypoxemia.

PFT: Not performed.

Chest radiograph: Lobar, peribronchial, and nodular infiltrates may be evidence of a fungal pneumonia.

Other data: Aspergillus antigen skin test.

CBC: Decrease in WBCs, neutrophils, and lymphocytes.

Sputum Gram stain: Gram-positive and -negative rods and yeasts may be present.

Sputum C&S: Presence of fungal organism. Aspiration via bronchoscopy is sometimes indicated if a sufficient sample cannot be obtained.

TREATMENT

- Amphotericin B and itraconazole are used to treat fungal infections. Other antibiotics may be indicated if multiple organisms are suspected.
- Oxygen therapy is used to alleviate hypoxemia. Antipyretics are used for fever. Adequacy of systemic hydration should also be assessed.

QUESTIONS FREQUENTLY ASKED BY PATIENT OR CAREGIVER

1. The doctor told me about treatment for the fungus, but the treatment sounds worse than the disease. Do I really need the treatment?

Most people do not need treatment for fungus infections; however, in some cases, the fungus can be life threatening. So, if your physician recommends treatment, he or she must be especially concerned about you and your case. The two most common forms of treatment are amphotericin B and fluconazole/itraconazole. Amphotericin B is the gold standard, "tried-and-true" treatment, but it requires 4 hours of IV infusions several times per week and can cause fever, chills, malaise, and kidney injury. Fluconazole and itraconazole have few side effects and suppress fungus infections well but are not as good at curing infections as amphotericin B is. They may require months or years of treatment.

2. When my mother had TB, they put her in quarantine for 2 months. But no one has talked to me about isolation. Shouldn't I wear a mask to avoid spreading infection?

No. Fungus organisms are infectious only in the wild state while living in the soil. The form of the organism changes in the body and becomes noncontagious. For that reason, you will not need isolation. The most widely recognized instance of person-to-person spread of a fungus infection occurred at Riverside General Hospital in California. A motorcycle accident victim's leg cast became infected with valley fever. Many of the hospital workers associated with the patient became ill with valley fever. This was unusual because the motorcycle accident victim was not known to have valley fever, but the cast had allowed the fungus to grow as a wild type.

3. Is treatment going to be expensive?

Amphotericin B is not very expensive to purchase, but IV delivery for several hours several times a week for several months becomes expensive. Fluconazole and itraconazole are very expensive to purchase and must be used for months to years. Fortunately, most insurance companies pay for the medication if serious infection is documented by a physician.

4. I was told that my chest radiograph was normal, but the physician is recommending treatment for the fungus infection. Why don't they leave me alone?

Fungus infections most commonly affect the lungs, but they can affect many other areas of the body. Widespread evidence of fungus infection requires treatment even though the lungs have been spared.

5. Where did I get this fungal infection?

Fungus is common in the soil in many parts of the country. West Texas, Arizona, and California have coccioidomycosis, and the Ohio River Valley has histoplasmosis. If you were recently in one of these areas, you may have become infected from exposure to the soil or dust.

6. If it is so common, how did I catch the fungus when everyone else has equal opportunity and did not become infected with the fungus?

Exposure is the first requirement for infection: windy, dusty days in the West expose more people to cocci. Excavations in the Ohio River Valley expose more people to histoplasmosis. Anyone exposed to dust such as dirt bike riders, motorcyclists, or archaeologists and museum workers are at risk for fungal infections.

Poor resistance is the second requirement for infection. People of some ethnicities are more prone to serious valley fever infections than others, and people with compromised immune systems (e.g., those undergoing chemotherapy or having AIDS) are more prone to infection. You should talk to your doctor for more specific details on your case.

7. I drink a six pack during every sports game and I watch at least one game on television every night. Will that interfere with my treatment?

Yes, in two ways. The first problem is that heavy alcohol use decreases a person's resistance. The second problem is that heavy alcohol use makes a person's liver more susceptible to damage by fluconazole or itraconazole.

8. My doctor said I have a cavity in my lung. Shouldn't it be taken out?

Under most circumstances, a pulmonary cavity gradually gets smaller and less visible on the chest radiograph as the infection resolves. Surgery is usually unnecessary unless the cavity becomes complicated.

9. How do they know I have a fungal infection?

The diagnosis is often suspected from your history presentation taken by your doctor. It is confirmed by a specimen sent to the laboratory.

10. What does the fungus do to my lungs?

The most common effects are early appearance of pneumonia and later changes such as scars or nodules in the lung that do no harm but appear on your chest radiograph. It would be a good idea for you to get an exact size, shape, and location of any nodules described in your medical record for future reference. Physicians who look at your chest radiograph in the future can tell if the nodule is changing and represents new pathology or not.

References

Braun, SR, et al.: Concise Textbook of Pulmonary Medicine. Elsevier, New York, 1989.

Thomas, CL: Taber's Cyclopedic Medical Dictionary, 18th edition. FA Davis, Philadelphia, 1997.

Wilkins, RL, Dexter, JR: Respiratory Disease: A Case Study Approach to Patient Care, second edition. FA Davis, Philadelphia, 1998.

Chapter 20

Pulmonary Thromboembolic Disease

Pulmonary thromboembolism is defined as a blood clot lodged in the pulmonary vasculature that typically originates in the deep veins of the lower extremities or pelvic area. The size of the clot determines the degree of disturbance in lung function.

KEY TERMS

angiography—visualization of the pulmonary vasculature by radiography after injecting radiopaque contrast medium into the pulmonary arteries

anticoagulation—the process of inhibiting blood from clotting

heparin—a medication used to reduce the formation of blood clots

infarction (pulmonary)—death of a portion of the lung tissue because of a blood clot blocking circulation to the affected area

thrombus—blood clot

thrombosis—the formation of a blood clot

V/Q lung scan—a nuclear medicine examination in which a subject is injected with a radioactive isotope and also breathes a radioactive gas; the lungs are then scanned to determine any mismatches of ventilation to perfusion

EPIDEMIOLOGY

Not applicable.

ETIOLOGY

Three factors cause pulmonary thromboemboli:

1. Stasis of the blood (e.g., prolonged bed rest)
2. Hypercoagulability of the blood
3. Trauma to the blood vessels

CLINICAL FEATURES

The clinical features of the patient with a pulmonary embolism vary widely and depend on the size and number of clots lodged in the lung or lungs and the underlying health status of the patient.

Medical History

Can occur at any age but is most often seen in adults. Pulmonary embolism is nonspecific for ethnicity or gender.

Chief Complaints

Most patients complain of acute dyspnea, which may be transient. Other complaints that occur less often include pleuritic chest pain, cough, and leg swelling. Hemoptysis is rare. Fainting spells suggest a large pulmonary embolus that is compromising blood flow to the left ventricle and subsequent cardiac output.

Past Medical History

May be positive for trauma or long-term bed rest (stasis).

Family History

Noncontributory.

Occupational and Social History

Not applicable.

Physical Examination

The physical examination findings vary widely depending on the size of the clot(s) in the lungs and the previous condition of the pulmonary system.

Respiratory rate and heart rate are often increased. BP is usually normal but may be reduced if the clot is large enough to compromise blood flow return to the left side of the heart. A mild fever may be present.

HEENT: JVD may be present if the clot is large.

Chest: Often normal but may reveal a localized area of crackles and wheezing if the clot is large enough to damage lung tissue. A loud P-2 may be present in those with pulmonary hypertension. A pleural friction rub is rarely present.

Hemodynamics and Laboratory Data

CVP and PAP: are usually elevated.

PCWP: Normal or low. A reduced PCWP suggests that blood flow to the left side of the heart is compromised.

Chest radiograph: Often normal but may show a localized area of poor perfusion. Signs of volume loss and pleural effusion may be seen in rare cases.

V/Q scans: Show areas of poor perfusion but normal ventilation if pulmonary emboli are present.

ABG: Usually show mild to moderate hypoxemia with respiratory alkalosis.

Pulmonary angiography is the definitive test and demonstrates the clot or clots.

CBC: Often normal unless an underlying infection is present.

TREATMENT

The goals of treatment are twofold:

1. Treat the current vascular occlusion and the resulting hemodynamic consequences
2. Prevent future clots from forming

Anticoagulant therapy using heparin is the most common initial treatment. This helps prevent additional clots but does little to alter the current clots in the lung.

Thrombolytic agents such as streptokinase can be used in severe cases to break up the current clots but are associated with potential side effects. They are contraindicated in patients who have recently had surgery because they may induce bleeding.

Oxygen therapy is often needed to maintain the PaO_2 in the 80 to 100 mm HG range. This can usually be accomplished with nasal cannula at low flows unless the pulmonary emboli are many or large.

Figure 20–1 outlines the diagnosis and treatment of pulmonary embolism.

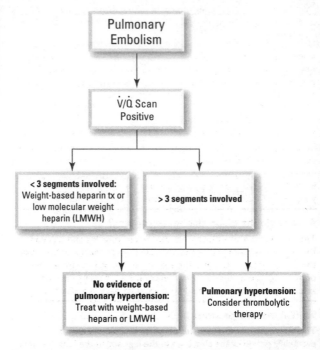

Figure 20–1. *Assessment and treatment of pulmonary embolism.*

QUESTIONS FREQUENTLY ASKED BY PATIENT OR CAREGIVER

1. Why am I so short of breath?

A pulmonary embolus blocks blood flow to part of the lung, so air going to that part of the lung does not provide oxygen to the blood and is thus wasted. In addition to wasted ventilation, blood clots release many chemicals that cause bronchospasm and shortness of breath.

2. Where did the blood clot come from?

Most blood clots are formed in leg veins. They break off from the leg veins and travel through the bloodstream to the heart, through the heart, and into the lung. The small blood vessels in the lung catch the clot and prevent it from going any further. Another possible site of origin for blood clots in the lung is the right heart.

3. Why did I get the clot?

The three major causes of blood clot formation are stasis, hypercoagulability, and vein wall injury. Approximately 5% of the U.S. population has a genetic defect that makes them more likely to develop clots. Long trips, illness, or paralysis can cause stasis of blood in the legs. Surgery or injury can damage the lining of the veins in your leg and make them more likely to attract clot formation.

4. How did the blood clot get to my lung?

The blood clot broke loose from the vein in your leg and traveled through the veins of your leg to the vein in your chest and from that through your heart and into the vein in your lung. The smaller vessels of the lung "catch" the clot and prevent it from passing into the arterial system, where it could do greater damage like a stroke.

5. Will the clot go away?

The body has potent clotbuster enzymes that almost always eventually get rid of the clot, both in the legs and in the lung. It is very uncommon for a clot to be left in the lung; it is more common for a clot to be left in the leg. If the clot is left in the leg, the body will form new little blood vessels right through the clot. In most cases, treatment for clots is designed to prevent new clot formation until the old clots can be removed or stabilized with new blood vessels growing through it.

6. What are the common forms of treatment for clots?

Classical treatment for blood clots has been heparin given either IV or subcutaneous injection for about 7 days followed by 6 days of treatment with coumadin pills.

7. Are there new forms of treatment for clots?

Two new forms of treatment have become more popular over the past 5 years. The first form of treatment is the "clotbuster" class of medications that you may have heard about as a treatment for heart attack. The advantages of clotbuster drugs are that they remove clot quickly and efficiently. The disadvantages of clotbuster drugs are that they only work on fresh clots and they can cause bleeding that may be serious or fatal. The second form of treatment is related to heparin but is a more purified form of heparin called LMWH. LMWH does not require as careful monitoring as heparin and is slightly more effective than heparin with slightly lower risk of bleeding than associated with heparin. The major advantage of LMWH is that it allows treatment for some clots at home rather than in the hospital. It is relatively expensive but is much less expensive than the day in the hospital. You should consult your physician to identify which treatment is best in your specific case.

8. I want the "clotbuster drug." Please arrange for me to get it!

Decisions about treatment options associated with risks as severe as the clotbuster drugs should be made only after extensive discussions with your physician. If your symptoms have been present for less than 5 days and you have no known bleeding risks, then ask your nurse to contact your physician for his advice about treatment with the clotbuster drug.

9. Why am I stuck in the hospital? I want to be treated at home.

The most respected studies show that many people with blood clots in their legs can be treated at home. This would require a home health nurse to provide LMWH shots at home and would also require someone at home with you to provide for your needs during the first week. Ask your doctor when it would be safe for you to go home.

10. This is my third admission to the hospital with a blood clot in my leg. How can I stop this inconvenience?

People with recurrent clots usually have a high risk for clot formation, either because they have very coagulable blood or very damaged veins. People with these problems are most often treated with lifetime anticoagulation with coumadin. Your doctor can give you advice about the risks of lifetime treatment with coumadin compared with the risks of recurrent blood clots in your legs.

11. Will I cough up this blood clot out of my lungs?

No. It will dissolve in the pulmonary blood vessels in most cases. However, you may cough up a little blood if the clot is large enough to damage a major portion of the lung.

12. Will these blood clots affect my heart?

No. The clots usually pass through the heart without causing any damage or changes to the heart.

Reference

Wilkins, RL, Dexter, JR: Respiratory Disease: A Case Study Approach to Patient Care, second edition. FA Davis, Philadelphia, 1998.

Chapter 21

Respiratory Distress Syndrome in the Newborn

RDS is primarily seen in premature infants and is characterized by surfactant deficiency and immature anatomic development of the lungs.

KEY TERMS

acrocyanosis–cyanosis of the extremities

hyaline membrane disease–presence of a proteinaceous membrane (hyaline) as a result of lung injury

PDA–failure to close the ductus arteriosus, a fetal heart structure, after birth; the opening allows a shunting between pulmonary and systemic circulations

EPIDEMIOLOGY

Newborns born before 38 weeks gestation are at risk. White male infants are at highest risk, as are infants younger than 29 weeks gestational age and low birth weight (<1500 g). The peak incidence is 60% in 28- to 30-week gestational age infants.

ETIOLOGY

Incidence increased with prematurity, second-born twin, perinatal asphyxia, cesarean section without labor, maternal history of previous RDS birth, and gestational diabetes.

CLINICAL FEATURES

Medical History

Chief Complaint

Evidence of respiratory distress soon after delivery. Differential diagnosis is pneumonia or transient tachypnea.

History of Present Illness

Progressive worsening of respiratory distress after birth.

Past Medical History

Prematurity, low birth weight, cesarean section, second-born twin, maternal history for diabetes.

Family History

Sibling born with RDS.

Occupational and Social History

Noncontributory. Access to prenatal care during pregnancy may help in screening for potential RDS birth.

Physical Examination

Central cyanosis.

Vital signs: Tachycardia with tachypnea. Breathing pattern may be irregular with apneic periods.

Sensorium: Normal.

HEENT: Presence of flaring nostrils, audible grunting.

Neck: Normal.

Chest: PDA.

Inspection: Subcostal and intercostal retractions.

Auscultation: Decreased with bilateral crackles.

Abdomen: Normal.

Extremities: Pallor or cyanosis.

Laboratory Data

ABG: Hypoxemia. Respiratory acidosis may not be present until the disease progresses.

PFT: Not routinely performed, but show decreased volumes and decreased compliance.

Chest radiography: Low-volume with diffuse granular (ground-glass) appearance. Air bronchograms may be present. High-volume radiography may suggest pneumonia.

Other data: Cultures to differentiate pneumonia.

TREATMENT

- Prevention by prenatal administration of I.V. corticosteroids to the mother
- Exogenous surfactant and oxygen
- CPAP and mechanical ventilation in cases of ventilatory failure
- Prostaglandin inhibitor (indomethacin) to hasten closure of the PDA

QUESTIONS FREQUENTLY ASKED BY PATIENT OR CAREGIVER

1. What does surfactant do?

Surfactant decreases the surface tension of the alveoli. This prevents collapse of the lung during expiration and decreases the infant's work during inspiration. Surfactant also dries out the airways.

2. Is this disease fatal?

Although some infants might die from this disease, it is usually not fatal. You should ask your baby's doctor about your baby's prognosis.

3. Will my child have long-term lung damage?

Some infants might develop chronic lung disease or bronchopulmonary dysplasia as a complication of RDS and mechanical ventilation. Most infants recover and have completely normal lungs. Infants who are extremely immature are at greatest risk. You should ask your baby's doctor about your baby's prognosis.

4. Are there any other long-term complications?

Other complications are related to the maturity of your infant, not to whether your infant has RDS. You should ask your baby's doctor about your baby's prognosis.

5. Will my child have any learning disabilities?

It is possible that your child might have learning disabilities. These are more likely related to problems associated with being premature than with having RDS.

6. If I have any more children, will they get RDS as well?

Subsequent children will develop RDS only if they are born prematurely. There is a familial tendency that is related to the severity of RDS. If a family has a preterm infant who has severe RDS, a subsequent preterm infant who has RDS would probably also have severe disease.

7. Is there anything I could have done during my pregnancy to have prevented this?

No. Obstetricians can give a mother who is in preterm labor medications (steroids) to accelerate the maturation of the infant's lungs.

8. Is it hereditary?

RDS is not hereditary. It is related to the maturity of the lung.

9. Will the child require special care at home?

If your child does not have any complications, he or she will not require any special care at home.

10. Is my child at greater risk of SIDS?

RDS does not increase the risk of SIDS. There is a slightly greater risk of SIDS in preterm infants and in infants who have chronic lung disease. You should ask your baby's doctor about your baby's prognosis.

Reference

Wilkins, RL, and Dexter, JR: Respiratory Disease: A Case Study Approach to Patient Care, second edition. FA Davis, Philadelphia, 1998.

Chapter 22

Respiratory Syncytial Virus

Respiratory syncytial virus is a virus that causes neighboring cells to form a conglomerate or syncytium. Infection of the respiratory tract with RSV is common in children and may lead to severe symptoms of cough, congestion, and pneumonia.

KEY TERMS

ribavirin–generic name for the antiviral medication used to treat patients with RSV

SPAG–device used to create small, consistent particles to maximize penetration and deposition of ribavirin

EPIDEMIOLOGY

Most frequent childhood pathogen. Leading cause of bronchiolitis and pneumonia in children; rare in children younger than age 4 months. RSV causes 90,000 hospitalizations and 4500 deaths a year.

ETIOLOGY

Contact with secretions or aerosolized secretions of an individual with coldlike symptoms. More common in midwinter and early spring. The virus has an incubation period of 2 to 8 days.

CLINICAL FEATURES

Vary with age and severity.

Medical History
Chief Complaints
Runny nose, sore throat, cough, low-grade temperature.

History of Present Illness

Prior exposure to sibling or parent with coldlike symptoms with specific attention to time of year.

Past Medical History

Patients with cystic fibrosis, congenital heart disease, bronchopulmonary dysplasia, or immunodeficiencies are at higher risk for severe disease.

Family History

Noncontributory.

Occupational and Social History

Children in day care are at higher risk.

Physical Examination

Vital Signs: Tachypnea, tachycardia, fever.

Sensorium: Alert.

HEENT: Grunting, nasal flaring with discharge, erythematous tympanic membranes.

Neck: Inspiratory stridor is common.

Chest:

Inspection: Costal and substernal retractions.

Palpation: Tactile fremitus.

Percussion: Normal.

Auscultation: I/E crackles, wheezing.

Abdomen: Normal.

Extremities: Normal.

Laboratory Data

ABG: Mild hypoxemia.

PFT: Not indicated.

Chest radiography: Hyperinflation and infiltrates are common.

Other data:

CBC: Normal.

C&S: Positive RSV culture results from nasal lavage or nasopharyngeal aspirate.

TREATMENT

Patients are treated with oxygen and mechanical ventilation. Ribavirin via SPAG, once the treatment of choice, is now a "drug that may be considered," according to the American Academy of Pediatrics. Newer drugs include RespiGam, an immune globulin administered I.V., and Palivizumab (Synagis), an antibody to provide passive immunity administered IM.

QUESTIONS FREQUENTLY ASKED BY PATIENT OR CAREGIVER

1. What is RSV?

"RSV" stands for "respiratory syncytial virus," the leading cause of lower respiratory tract infections in infants and young children. All children get RSV infections, and reinfections occur throughout life.

2. How did my child get RSV?

RSV spreads easily from person to person through respiratory secretions. Spread within families is very high.

3. Will my child get RSV again?

Yes. Reinfections occur throughout life. Reinfection illnesses are generally mild.

4. Can RSV infection be prevented?

No. Attempts to develop a vaccine have not yet been effective, and immunity after an infection is transient and imperfect.

5. How long will my child be in the hospital?

The average duration of hospitalization for previously healthy infants is 4 to 7 days; full recovery may take up to 2 weeks.

6. Will RSV weaken my child's lungs and make him or her more susceptible to pneumonia in the future?

The vast majority of children recover completely. A few children appear to be more susceptible to subsequent respiratory problems. You should ask your child's doctor if he or she thinks your child will have future problems.

7. Why are you prescribing bronchodilators for my child? I thought they were used for patients with asthma.

There is a similarity of symptoms and signs of RSV broncholitis and asthma. In addition, bronchospasm has been shown to be present in children with RSV, in many cases. The bronchodilators make it easier for your child to breathe.

8. Does RSV infection cause asthma?

There is no clear evidence suggesting that RSV infection causes asthma. However, some children may have recurrent wheezing episodes after their RSV infection. You should ask your doctor if your child is one of these children.

9. Can RSV be serious?

Yes. The most serious infections occur in newborns and infants and those who have other complicating or underlying conditions, such as congenital heart disease, lung disease, or prematurity.

10. Why isn't the doctor prescribing antibiotics?

RSV is a viral infection that doesn't respond to antibiotics.

11. Why isn't the doctor prescribing steroids?

Corticosteroids do not change the acute course of RSV bronchiolitis in previously healthy infants without underlying disease.

12. Why did my baby stop breathing? Will he or she be able to breathe normally after this RSV is gone?

Apnea is a striking complication that occurs in a small percent of infants hospitalized with RSV. The reasons for apnea in RSV infections are not understood. Apnea resolves in 48 to 72 hours, and most often does not recur.

References

American Academy of Pediatrics Committee on Infectious Diseases: Reassessment of the indications for ribavirin therapy in respiratory syncytial virus. *Pediatrics* 1996, 97:137–140.

Darville, T, and Yamauchi, T: Respiratory syncytial virus. *Pediatr Review* 1998, 19:55–61.

Everard, ML: What link between early respiratory viral infections and atopic asthma? *Lancet* 1999, 354:527–528.

Hall, CB: Respiratory syncytial virus: A continuing culprit and conundrum. *J Pediatr* 1999, 135:S2–S7.

Kellne, JD, et al: Efficacy of bronchodilator therapy in bronchiolitis. *Arch Pediatr Adolesc Med* 1996, 150:1166–1172.

Probe, CG, and Sullender, WM: Advances in prevention of respiratory syncytial virus infections. *J Pediatr* 1999, 135:546–558.

Wilkins, RL, and Dexter, JR: Respiratory Disease: A Case Study Approach to Patient Care, second edition. FA Davis, Philadelphia, 1998.

Chapter 23

Shock

Shock is an inadequate perfusion of the vital organs that leads to tissue hypoxia. It is a common cause of death in patients in the ICU and has a large variety of causes. Shock can occur at any age and is nonspecific to gender or ethnicity.

KEY TERMS

afterload–the resistance to blood flow out of the ventricle

cardiac index–cardiac output divided by body surface area

cardiac output–the volume of blood pumped each minute by the left ventricle

hypovolemic shock–shock caused by low blood volume

inotrope–medication that affects the heart's contractility

perfusion–the movement of blood into a specific vascular space

preload–the volume of blood in the ventricle just before contraction

septic shock–shock caused by severe infection and loss of vascular tone

stroke volume–the volume of blood ejected by the ventricle with each contraction

ETIOLOGY

There are three basic causes of shock:

1. Loss of circulating blood volume
2. Loss of vascular tone (e.g., septic shock)
3. Loss of contractility (e.g., poor pumping ability)

CLINICAL FEATURES

Medical History

Chief Complaints

Patient may not be alert, but if he or she is, complains of dizziness, weakness, and dyspnea.

History of Present Illness

May have experienced recent onset of chest pain if coronary artery disease is present. May have recent history of trauma if hypovolemic shock is present. History of infection is present when sepsis is the cause.

Past Medical History

Often positive for heart disease in patients with coronary artery disease. The history may be negative otherwise.

Family History

Noncontributory.

Occupational and Social History

Noncontributory.

Physical Examination

Patients with shock are usually confused, disoriented, or comatose. BP is reduced below 90/60 mm Hg. Heart and respiratory rate are usually increased.

HEENT: Noncontributory.

Chest: Fine crackles in the bases are common when heart failure is the cause of the shock. Heart sounds are often soft and distant. Breathing is rapid and shallow.

Abdomen: Noncontributory.

Extremities: Often cool to touch, and capillary refill is greater than 3 seconds except in patients with septic shock; cyanosis may also be seen. Peripheral pulses are weak.

Laboratory Data

CBC: Shows elevated WBC if infection is present, as in septic shock.

ECG: May show tachycardia with elevated or depressed ST segments and large Q waves if ischemic heart disease is the cause.

Chest radiograph: Often shows a large heart and pulmonary edema if left ventricular failure is the cause. If HF is not the cause, the chest radiograph may be normal.

ABG: Often demonstrates hypoxemia with respiratory alkalosis at first but progresses to metabolic acidosis when the tissue hypoxia is severe. Anion gap elevates in such cases.

Urine output: Low (< 30 cc/h).

Hemodynamic monitoring: Demonstrates elevated PCWP in cases of HF but normal to low PCWP in those with septic shock. SVR is elevated in most cases of shock but is reduced in those with septic shock.

TREATMENT

- Most patients in severe shock require oxygen therapy at high FIO_2s and intubation to protect and maintain an airway.
- Mechanical ventilation is possible with PEEP if refractory hypoxemia is present. Mechanical ventilation allows the respiratory muscles to rest and reduces oxygen consumption.
- Replacement of blood volume is important when hypovolemic shock is present.
- Appropriate antibiotics are needed when sepsis is occurring.

QUESTIONS FREQUENTLY ASKED BY PATIENT OR CAREGIVER

1. The doctor says my spouse is in shock. What does he mean?

Shock is a condition in which the body is not getting enough blood to all the areas of the body. Many patients with shock have low BPs, but this is not necessary.

2. Shock sounds serious. Is it?

Yes, shock can be a very serious condition. Often, if the shock is mild and treatment is promptly started, the shock completely stops.

3. Is shock like HF?

In some instances, shock is caused by HF. In many other cases, a different problem, such as bleeding, a severe infection, or a bad allergic reaction, can cause shock.

4. My husband has a severe infection. The doctors have given him so much IV fluid that he is very swollen. Do they have to give him so much?

When someone has severe shock, he or she must get many types of IV fluids. Sometimes the amount of fluid needed is significant. Some of this fluid leaks into the tissue and is seen as swelling. When your husband recovers, the swelling in his hands and other tissues will completely resolve.

5. The doctor just put a special catheter into my son to monitor his shock. I think the doctor called it a "swan cats" catheter. What does this catheter tell you?

This catheter, called the Swan-Ganz catheter, monitors the performance of the heart as well as the amount of fluids he needs. This kind of catheter is helpful in showing your son's doctor what kind of shock your son has. It may help the doctor tailor therapy to your son's needs.

6. (Wife at her husband's bedside. The husband is being treated for cardiogenic shock.) His hands are so cold. Why does this happen?

The cold hands are just a part of the disease process. When his heart function improves, his hands will become warmer and have better color.

7. My wife is so sick. Can she make it?

It is impossible to tell the future with any confidence when we are talking about the human body. Your wife's doctor may be able to give you an idea of what the likelihood is that your wife will recover completely.

8. All this high-tech treatment and she is still like this. She would never want to be this way. Can't someone make the doctor stop all this and let her go with some dignity?

You need to raise these concerns with the doctor. No one wants her to suffer unnecessarily or against her wishes. If she did not wish to be kept alive on machines, the doctor needs to know this. Should I page the doctor for you?

9. Can my husband hear me even though he does not respond to my voice?

We do not know for sure, but it doesn't hurt to assume that he can.

10. Can this shock cause brain damage to my husband?

Brain damage does not usually occur, but you should talk to your doctor about this more if you have concerns about your husband's case.

Reference

Wilkins, RL, and Dexter, JR: Respiratory Disease: A Case Study Approach to Patient Care, second edition. FA Davis, Philadelphia, 1998.

Chapter 24

Sleep Apnea

Obstructive sleep apnea (OSA) is respiratory effort without airflow caused by blockage or increased resistance in the upper airway. It is most often seen in obese males with narrowing of the upper airway caused by redundant tissue and a large tongue.

KEY TERMS

central sleep apnea–cessation of airflow caused by temporary loss of respiratory effort

epoch–arbitrary 30-second period used for staging sleep when interpreting a sleep study

hypopnea–period of 50% decrease of thoracoabdominal movement lasting 10 seconds during sleep

macroglossia–condition in which the tongue is larger than normal

micrognathia–condition in which the mandible is structurally small

mixed sleep apnea–combination of obstructive and central apnea

multiple sleep latency test–a series of daytime naps in which a patient is put to bed and the amount of time it takes for the patient to fall asleep is documented; it is an objective way to measure daytime sleepiness

NREM and REM sleep–stages of sleep with distinctive breathing patterns

respiratory disturbance index–also called the apnea/hypopnea index, it equals the number of events/sleep time in hours; index > 5 is abnormal (30 events in 6 hours of sleep) and is clinically significant at 20

sleep apnea–cessation of breathing for at least 10 seconds during sleep

EPIDEMIOLOGY

Approximately 4% of women and 9% of men have significant OSA.

ETIOLOGY

Obesity, structural abnormalities such as micrognathia and macroglossia, or anatomic narrowing of the upper airway.

CLINICAL FEATURES

The patient is usually seen by a doctor at the insistence of the bed partner.

Medical History

Chief Complaints

Excessive daytime sleepiness, snoring, decreased concentration, bed wetting, or apneic events reported by the bed partner.

History of Present Illness

The patient may report falling asleep while driving, disruption of work or social life, memory loss, mood changes, or morning headache.

Past Medical History

Noncontributory.

Family History

Noncontributory.

Occupational and Social History

Noncontributory.

Physical Examination

May be obese.

Vital Signs: Possibly hypertensive.

Sensorium: Normal but may appear fatigued.

HEENT: Micrognathia, macroglossia, large uvula, narrow posterior pharynx.

Neck: Short, thick neck; JVD with cor pulmonale.

Chest:

Inspection: Normal.

Palpation: Normal.

Percussion: Normal.

Auscultation: Normal.

Abdomen: Normal or obese.

Extremities: Edema in lower extremities if cor pulmonale is present.

Laboratory Data

ABG: Normal in most individuals during daytime; possible hypercapnia and hypoxemia in obese individuals.

PFT: Normal but possible "sawtooth" pattern in expiratory limb of the flow-volume loop.

Chest Radiography: Normal or evidence of pulmonary hypertension.

Other data: Polysomnogram, MSLT.

TREATMENT

- Weight loss, avoidance of alcohol, and sedatives for mild cases
- CPAP for moderate to severe disease; must monitor for patient compliance
- UPPP or dental appliances for those patients not responding to CPAP

Figure 24–1 outlines the assessment and treatment of obstructive sleep apnea.

QUESTIONS FREQUENTLY ASKED BY PATIENT OR CAREGIVER

1. Is it safe to drive my car if I have sleep apnea?

Not if you are experiencing excessive daytime sleepiness. To avoid injury, consult with your doctor about this before you attempt to drive or perform any function that requires concentration.

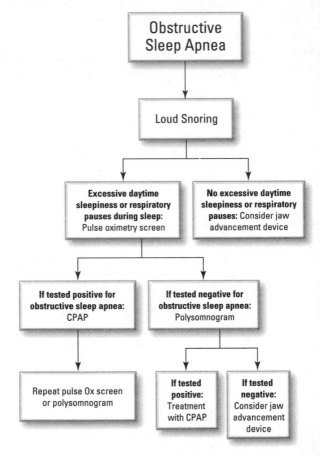

Figure 24–1. *Assessment and treatment of obstructive sleep apnea.*

2. Does surgery help for my condition?

Some patients with OSA respond well to surgical treatment, but CPAP is usually more effective and is associated with fewer side effects.

3. Can I drink alcohol at bedtime?

No. Alcohol consumption increases the severity of the problem.

4. Can I die from sleep apnea?

The death rate from OSA is very low, but OSA is associated with increased hypertensive heart disease, impotence, and auto accidents. Your overall quality of life can be improved significantly with treatment.

5. Does my partner have to sleep in a separate room?

No. The CPAP machine makes very little noise and will cure the snoring.

6. Is there any medication I should take?

Not really, but a nasal decongestant may prove helpful when your nose is plugged because of a cold.

7. Is there any medication I should avoid?

Sleeping pills and sedatives should be avoided.

8. What are the side effects from the CPAP machine?

Some patients experience a pressure sore on the bridge of their nose from the mask if it is not adjusted correctly. You may also notice a dry throat or irritation from an air leak. These are relatively minor and can be corrected in most cases.

9. Will I have this condition for the rest of my life?

Many people with OSA no longer need the CPAP machine when they reach their ideal body weight.

10. Will it get worse?

The symptoms may increase with weight gain or nasal congestion.

11. How did I get this problem?

OSA is most often caused by abnormalities that decrease the size of the opening in the upper airway. People who are overweight, have a large tongue, large tonsils, short thick neck, or a receding lower jaw are prone to developing the problem.

12. How about laser surgery? Does that work?

You can consult with your physician, but it appears that most studies on laser surgery are showing similar results as the regular surgery to remove redundant tissue. The laser surgery may not completely resolve the problem, and symptoms often return with time after the surgery.

Reference

Wilkins, RL, and Dexter, JR: Respiratory Disease: A Case Study Approach to Patient Care, second edition. FA Davis, Philadelphia, 1998.

Chapter 25

Smoke Inhalation and Burns

Smoke inhalation and burns represent serious threats to a patient's life. The most immediate threat is from CO poisoning, which leads to tissue hypoxia. Serious burns represent a threat to life days after the burn caused by infection and other complications.

KEY TERMS

anaerobic metabolism–metabolism without oxygen

CO poisoning–a buildup of CO in the blood that causes toxic symptoms

carboxyhemoglobin–hemoglobin bound with CO

catabolic hypermetabolism–metabolism in which the body breaks down more complex proteins into more simple substances

escharotomy–surgical incisions on a severely burned chest wall to remove scabs and make chest movement and breathing easier

flashover–a wall of fire extending down from the ceiling and billowing out of open doors or windows

hydrogen cyanide–a poisonous gas that blocks the tissues from using oxygen

EPIDEMIOLOGY

More than 23 million fires are reported in the U.S. each year. They are responsible for 28,000 injuries and approximately 5000 deaths each year.

CLINICAL FEATURES

The clinical features vary widely, depending on the extent of the burns and the amount of smoke inhaled. In addition, the time elapsed from exposure to the fire is a major factor in determining the clinical findings.

Medical History

Chief Complaints

Dyspnea, cough, headache, pain from burns.

History of Present Illness

Recent exposure to smoke, fire, or both in an enclosed building.

Past Medical History

Noncontributory.

Family History

Noncontributory.

Occupational and Social History

Noncontributory.

Physical Examination

Vital signs: Tachycardia and tachypnea are frequently present. Sensorium is abnormal if CO poisoning is present.

HEENT: Should be inspected for evidence of burns or exposure to smoke. Specifically, look for soot in the mouth or nose and singed nasal or facial hair.

Neck: May be normal or stridor may be present if the upper airway has been exposed to the extreme heat.

Chest: May be normal initially, but progressive abnormalities are common. Crackles and wheezes may be heard when the lower airways become involved.

Abdomen: Noncontributory.

Extremities: Often show evidence of burns.

Laboratory Data

The chest radiography and clinical laboratory data are often normal during the initial work-up of the patient. Later, the CBC may show leukocytosis with infection, and the chest radiography may demonstrate evidence of pneumonia and atelectasis if the fire has damaged the lower airway.

Pulse oximetry is of no value because it reads CO as oxygen on the hemoglobin.

ABG may be normal or demonstrate metabolic acidosis if anaerobic metabolism has been occurring.

TREATMENT

The goals of treatment are:

- Achieve and maintain a patent airway.
- Provide adequate oxygenation and ventilation.
- Maintain hemodynamic stability.
- Maintain acid–base balance.
- Monitor the patient carefully for signs of infection and respiratory failure.

Methods

- Signs of upper airway injury (e.g., stridor, cough, sooty sputum) suggest the need for intubation.
- Mechanical ventilation with PEEP may be needed at some point if respiratory failure ensues.
- High FIO_2 is needed if CO poisoning is present. Hyperbaric oxygen therapy is useful for more severe forms of CO poisoning.
- Bronchial hygiene techniques are often needed in the course of recovery if the fire has damaged the lower airways.
- Appropriate intake of nutrition and fluids is important over the course of recovery.
- Antibiotics are needed when infection is present.

QUESTIONS FREQUENTLY ASKED BY PATIENT OR CAREGIVER

1. Why is breathing smoke so harmful?

Smoke is composed of more than 1000 poisonous chemicals. The exact mixture in any fire depends on the substances burning and the amount of oxygen available to assist with the burning. One of the common and harmful gases produced by fire is CO. It binds very tightly to the hemoglobin in your blood and prevents adequate oxygenation of your body.

2. Why is oxygen therapy needed, and what is hyperbaric oxygen therapy?

Oxygen helps in two ways. It helps "wash" the CO off the hemoglobin and it provides the much-needed oxygen that the body is lacking because of the smoke inhalation. Using hyperbaric oxygen therapy increases the speed at which the CO is washed off the hemoglobin, so tissue oxygenation is returned to normal much faster. For example, CO has a half-life in the blood of about 300 minutes on room air but only 30 minutes with hyperbaric oxygen therapy.

3. Why is my voice hoarse and why can't I talk loudly?

Inhalation of smoke and hot air can damage the vocal cords and result in hoarseness. This problem should clear up in time. Consult your doctor for more details.

4. Why do I have such a terrible headache?

One of the gases given off during a fire is CO. High levels of CO in the blood can cause a severe headache. This should clear with treatment and time. Be sure to tell your doctor if you hit your head during the fire or rescue.

5. Why do you want to stick me in the wrist to draw arterial blood?

Arterial blood provides information about the condition of your lungs and how well they are functioning with gas exchange. Venous blood only tells us what oxygen is left over after metabolism. The arterial blood also can be tested with a co-oximeter that will test for poisoning. A small artery in the wrist is the safest place to get arterial blood.

6. I have never had asthma or bronchitis before, but now I can't stop coughing and wheezing. What is happening?

The smoke causes intense irritation of the small airways in the lungs. People with normal lungs often have persistent cough and wheezing for weeks after the original insult. People with sensitive airways are even more prone to bronchospasm after smoke exposure.

7. Why are there black specks in my sputum?

People who inhale smoke often also inhale soot. The soot collects in the sputum and is coughed out over time.

8. The doctor says he wants to put a tube in my trachea to protect my airway. What is that all about?

One of the most dangerous problems that can occur after serious smoke inhalation and burns is damage and inflammation to the upper airway. If this damage is significant, the airway can swell and can even cause very difficult breathing. The tube is only temporary to make sure you can breathe. It will be removed when the danger of airway swelling is over in a few days.

9. Why does my doctor want to do a bronchoscopy on me? Does it hurt?

The doctor wants to visualize the exact extent of the damage caused by the inhalation of smoke and hot air into your lungs. He can also use the bronchoscopy to clean out any foreign material that may be contributing to your breathing difficulties or that may cause problems later. The bronchoscopy procedure should not be painful.

10. Because I smoke cigarettes, will continuing this habit damage my lungs even more than usual?

It is very important that you not smoke for at least several weeks while your lungs are recovering from this injury. Your lungs are working hard to recover from the smoke inhalation and injury, and smoking cigarettes will only make things worse. In fact, this is a good time for you to consider entering a smoking cessation program.

Reference

Wilkins, RL, and Dexter, JR: Respiratory Disease: A Case Study Approach to Patient Care, second edition. FA Davis, Philadelphia, 1998.

Chapter 26

Tuberculosis

TB is an infection resulting from inhaled *Mycobacterium* particles. It was once a very common cause of death, but today the outlook is much brighter. It commonly occurs in patients with compromised immune systems, such as patients with AIDS.

KEY TERMS

BCG–vaccine containing a strain of *Mycobacterium bovis* used primarily as a preventive measure in developing countries

caseation–granuloma containing a cheesy center resulting from necrosis and parenchyma breakdown

Ghon complex–combination of initial lesion and affected lymph nodes

induration–an area of skin tissue that is hardened and often swollen

miliary TB–widespread infection in an organ system

Mantoux test–skin test using PPD

PPD–the substance used in an intradermal test for TB

primary TB–infection with the TB bacillus without the onset of symptoms and usually involving the middle or lower lobes

secondary TB–most common form of clinical TB; it results from an endogenous reinfection

Ziehl-Neelsen stain–a method for staining and identifying *Mycobacterium tuberculosis*

EPIDEMIOLOGY

Because of immigration and emergence of multidrug-resistant strains, TB is more common in immunosuppressed, malnourished, and institutionalized patients. One-third of the world's population is infected with it, and it is responsible for more than 30% of AIDS-related deaths.

ETIOLOGY

Transmitted by aerosolized droplets of *M. tuberculosis*. Primary infection results in positive skin test with little evidence of disease. Reactivation occurs in 10% of infected individuals.

CLINICAL FEATURES

Medical History

Chief Complaints

Fatigue, night sweats, chronic cough, hemoptysis, weight loss.

History of Present Illness

Slow development of symptoms over several weeks.

Past Medical History

Previous treatment for TB, BCG vaccination, prolonged pneumonias, uncontrolled diabetes, pleural effusions, malnutrition, alcoholism.

Family History

Relatives or friends with diagnosed TB.

Occupational and Social History

Occupational exposure to quartz or silica dust, recent foreign travel, contact with infected individuals or those at high risk.

Physical Examination

Not specific in making definitive diagnosis.

Vital Signs: Normal.

Sensorium: Normal.

HEENT: Normal.

Neck: Possible swollen lymph nodes.

Chest:

Inspection: Normal.

Palpation: Swollen lymph nodes.

Percussion: Dull.

Auscultation: Bronchial breath sounds, coarse crackles, wheezing.

Abdomen: Normal.

Extremities: Normal.

Laboratory Data

ABG: Normal or respiratory alkalosis with mild hypoxemia.

PFT: Not indicated.

Chest radiograph: Presence of cavitation, atelectasis, pleural effusion, and hilar lymphadenopathy.

Other data:

Sputum: Positive acid fast smear confirmed by positive culture results.

Skin testing: Positive reaction to PPD classified by the CDC as an induration of 5 mm or more.

TREATMENT

- Active infection: INH, rifampin, pyrazinamide, ethambutol, streptomycin
- Prophylactic: 6- to 9-month course of INH

QUESTIONS FREQUENTLY ASKED BY PATIENT OR CAREGIVER

1. Does a positive skin test mean I have TB?

Yes. But it is only infective to other people if the disease is active, as evidenced by a productive cough and a positive sputum TB smear result. Many people have a positive PPD result but are not infectious.

2. Can I get TB from shaking hands or other contact with infected individuals?

No. You can get TB only by breathing airborne droplets from an infective coughing or sneezing patient.

3. How often should I be tested after a positive PPD skin test?

After a PPD skin test has a positive result, it will always be positive, and no further skin testing is needed. A chest radiograph should be taken annually afterwards.

4. How often should I be tested after exposure to an infective person if my skin test was negative last year?

You should have one skin test immediately and then talk to your physician about prophylactic use of INH. You should have a follow-up skin test in 3 months to see whether the exposure caused an infection.

5. If I was exposed to a person with active TB, how long would it take for my skin test to become positive if I was infected?

A total of 6 to 8 weeks is the usual time.

6. Since I was diagnosed with TB, I frequently have to change my pajamas during the night because of heavy sweating. Why is this happening?

TB causes mild to moderate fevers that are often not noticed. The fever is often worse at night, and when the fever "breaks" during the night, there often is profuse sweating. Sweating is the body's attempt to deal with the fever and bring body temperature down.

7. Now that I have been diagnosed with active TB, how long will I need to take these medications?

Not long ago, the average treatment time was 18 months. Today, the average time the chemotherapy is needed is 6 to 9 months.

8. Will my lungs be permanently injured by the TB infection?

Not if the disease was diagnosed early and the correct treatment was given. If the disease was advanced at the time of diagnosis, some lung damage can occur. You should talk to your doctor about your specific case.

9. Why is my urine orange?

One of the medications used to treat TB (rifampin) makes all bodily secretions orange.

10. Why does everyone wear a mask when they enter my room?

Coughing causes small particles of mucus and TB germs to become airborne. These active TB organisms can remain airborne for hours and could be inhaled by others in the room. If they inhale the TB germs, they could also become infected.

11. What are the purple lights for?

Those are UV lights, and they kill the TB germs in the small droplets of mucus that you cough into the room. This helps reduce spreading of the disease.

12. Why do I need to take so many pills?

TB germs are naturally resistant to many antibiotics and can develop resistance to most antibiotics if they are not given in a combination program. It is also important that all the medications be taken as directed.

References

Braun, SR, *et al:* Concise Textbook of Pulmonary Medicine. Elsevier, New York, 1989.

Wilkins, RL, and Dexter, JR: Respiratory Disease: A Case Study Approach to Patient Care, second edition. FA Davis, Philadelphia, 1998.

Normal Laboratory Values*

Hoai N. Tran

ADULT

Arterial Blood Gases (ABGs)

pH	7.35–7.45
$Paco_2$	35–45 mm Hg
Pao_2	80–100 mm Hg
HCO_3^-	22–26 mEq/liter
Base excess (BE)	−2 to +2
Arterial saturation with oxygen (Sao_2)	>95 percent

Complete Blood Count (CBC)

Red blood cell (RBC) count	
Men	4.6–6.2 million/mm^3
Women	4.2–5.4 million/mm^3
Hemoglobin (Hb)	
Men	13.5–16.5 g/dL
Women	12.0–15.0 g/dL
Hematocrit (Hct)	
Men	40–54%
Women	38–47%
Erythrocyte index	
Mean cell volume (MCV)	80–96 μ^3

*Reproduced from Wilkins/Dexter: Respiratory Disease: A Case Study Approach to Patient Care. Ed 2. F.A. Davis Company, 1998.

Mean cell hemoglobin (MCH)	27–31 pg
Mean cell hemoglobin concentration (MCHC)	32–36%
White blood cell (WBC) count	4,500–10,000/mm³
Differential of WBCs	
Neutrophils	40–75%
Bands	0–6%
Eosinophils	0–6%
Basophils	0–1%
Lymphocytes	20–45%
Monocytes	2–10%
Platelet count	150,000–400,000/mm³

Chemistry

Na^+	137–147 mEq/liter
K^+	3.5–4.8 mEq/liter
Cl^-	98–105 mEq/liter
CO_2	25–33 mEq/liter
Blood urea nitrogen (BUN)	7–20 mg/dL
Creatine	0.7–1.3 mg/dL
Total protein	6.3–7.9 g/dL
Albumin	3.5–5.0 g/dL
Cholesterol	150–220 mg/dL
Glucose	70–105 mg/dL

Hemodynamic Values

Variable	Abbreviation	Normal
Cardiac output	Q̇T	4–8 liters/minute
Cardiac index	CI	2.5–4.0 liters/minute/m²
Stroke volume	SV	60–130 mL
Ejection fraction	EF	65–75%
Central venous pressure	CVP	0–6 mm Hg

Pulmonary artery pressure	PAP	25/10 mm Hg
Pulmonary capillary wedge pressure	PCWP	6–12 mm Hg
Systemic vascular resistance	SVR	900–1400 dynes/second/cm^5
Pulmonary vascular resistance	PVR	110–250 dynes/second/cm^5

Pulmonary Function Tests

Variable	Abbreviation	Normal
Forced vital capacity	FVC	>80% of predicted
Slow vital capacity	SVC	80–120% of predicted
Forced expiratory volume in 1 second	FEV_1	>80% of predicted
Forced expiratory volume in 1 second/Forced vital capacity	FEV_1/FVC	>75%
Forced expiratory flow	$FEF_{25-75°}$	>80% of predicted
Carbon monoxide diffusing capacity	D_{LCO}	25 mL CO/minute/mm Hg
Total lung capacity	TLC	6000 mL
Functional residual capacity	FRC	2400 mL
Residual volume	RV	1200 mL
Vital capacity	VC	4800 mL

Vital Signs	Normal Range
Temperature range	36.1–37.5°C
Heart rate	60–100/minute
Respiratory rate	12–20/minute
Blood pressure range	120/80 mm Hg
	Systolic 95–140 mm Hg
	Diastolic 60–90 mm Hg

CHILDREN (AGE 1 to 12 YEARS)

ABGs

Refer to adult values

CBC Tests

RBC count	3.8–5.5 million/mm^3
Hb	11–16 g/dL
Hct	31–43%
Erythrocyte index (refer to adult values)	
WBC count (refer to adult values)	
Differential of WBCs (refer to adult values)	

Chemistry

Na$^+$	135–145 mEq/liter
K$^+$	3.5–5.0 mEq/liter
Cl$^-$	100–106 mEq/liter
Ca^{++}	9.2–10.8 mg/dL
Mg^{++}	1.5–2.0 mEq/liter
Glucose	60–105 mg/dL

Hemodynamic Values

CI	3.5–4.5 liter/minute/m^2
CVP	2–6 mm Hg
PAP	30/8 mm Hg
PCWP	4–8 mm Hg

NEWBORN

ABG

pH	7.25–7.35
$PaCO_2$	26–40 mm Hg
PaO_2	50–70 mm Hg
HCO_3^-	17–23 mEq/liter
BE	-10 to -2

CBC Count

RBC count	4.8–7.1 million/mm³
Hb	14–24 g/dL
Hct	44–64%
Erythrocyte index	
MCV	96–108 μ^3
MCH	32–34 pg
MCHC	32–33%
WBC count	
Mean value	18,100/mm³
Range	9,000–30,0000/mm³
Lymphocytes	
Mean value	5,500/mm³
Range	2,000–11,000/mm³

Chemistry

Na^+	133–149 mEq/liter
K^-	5.3–6.4 mEq/liter
Cl^-	87–114 mEq/liter
CO_2	19–22 mEq/liter
Total protein	4.8–8.5 g/dL
Albumin	2.9–5.5 g/dL
Glucose	30–110 mg/dL

Hemodynamic Values

Cardiac output	
Newborn	0.8–1.0 liter/minute
6 months old	1.0–1.3 liters/minute
1 year old	1.3–1.5 liters/minute
CI	2.5–4.5 liters/minute/m^2
SV	
Newborn	5 mL
6 months old	10 mL
1 year old	13 mL

Vital Signs

Temperature range	36.1–37.5°C
Heart rate	100–160/minute
Respiratory rate	30–60/minute
Blood pressure	75/50 mm Hg